DEPARTMENT OF HEALTH AND SO

PESTICIDE POISONING

NOTES FOR THE GUIDANCE OF MEDICAL PRACTITIONERS

prepared jointly by
the Medical Panel of the Advisory Committee on Pesticides
and
The Toxicological Committee of the British Agrochemicals
Association Limited

LONDON: HER MAJESTY'S STATIONERY OFFICE

© Crown Copyright 1983
First published 1983

ISBN 0 11 320830 8

HER MAJESTY'S STATIONERY OFFICE
Government Bookshops
49 High Holborn, London WC1V 6HB
13a Castle Street, Edinburgh EH2 3AR
Brazennose Street, Manchester M60 8AS
Southey House, Wine Street, Bristol BS1 2BQ
258 Broad Street, Birmingham B1 2HE
80 Chichester Street, Belfast BT1 4JY

Government Publications are also available through booksellers

National Poisons Information Services

The National Poisons Information Services (NPIS) operate from 5 Centres (see below) to provide a 24-hour emergency service for information and advice on problems of acute toxicity and their treatment. Access to this service is generally restricted to the medical profession and the emergency services, and is not available to the public. In most instances, the initial enquiry will be answered by an information officer or a nurse but medical staff are always available for consultation. In addition, where appropriate, the Centres may be able to offer help with laboratory analyses for poisons and may be able to make referrals to other information services or expert opinions.

Another function of the NPIS is the monitoring of the incidence and severity of acute poisoning. The NPIS (London) would thus be grateful for information on any case of pesticide poisoning, even when the reporter does not need information. You are encouraged to make such reports which, in turn, increase the accuracy of the information available to enquirers.

Addresses and Telephone Numbers of the Centres:

LONDON:	Poisons Information Service New Cross Hospital Avonley Road LONDON SE14 5ER	Tel: 01 407 7600
EDINBURGH:	Poisons Information Service The Royal Infirmary Lauriston Place EDINBURGH E3	Tel: 031 229 2477
BELFAST:	Poisons Information Service Royal Victoria Hospital Grosvenor Road BELFAST B12 6BB	Tel: 0232 40503
DUBLIN:	Poisons Information Service Jervis Street Hospital DUBLIN 1	Tel: 0001 74 5588
CARDIFF:	Poisons Information Service Ambulance Headquarters Old Ty-Bronna Fairwater Road Fairwater CARDIFF CF5 3XP	Tel: 0222 569 200

Contents

National Poisons Information Services   page i

Introduction   1

Primary Treatment Measures   3

Index to Diagnosis and Treatment Section by Active Ingredients and Trade Names   5

Diagnosis and Treatment
1. Dinitrocompounds   33
2. Other uncouplers of Oxidative Phosphorylation   36
3. Organochlorine Compounds   38
4. Organophosphorus Compounds   40
5. Carbamates   45
6. Fluoroacetic Acid Derivatives   48
7. Organic Mercurials   50
8. Inorganic Mercurials   53
9. Arsenical Compounds   55
10. Pyrethrins and synthetic Pyrethroids   57
11. Bipyridylium Compounds   59
12. Phenoxyacetates and related Compounds   64
13. Organotin Compounds   66
14. Nicotine   67
15. Dithiocarbamate Fungicides   68
16. Triazine Herbicides   70
17. Chlorates   72
18. Anticoagulant Rodenticides   74
19. Fumigants   76
    - *a* Methyl Bromide   76
    - *b* Carbon Tetrachloride   79
    - *c* Ethylene Dichloride   81
    - *d* Ethylene Dibromide   82
    - *e* Chloropicrin   83
    - *f* Phosphine   84
    - *g* Cyanides   85

Appendices

I   The Health and Safety (Agriculture) (Poisonous Substances) Regulations, 1975 — 87

II Addresses and Telephone Numbers of Senior Employment Medical Advisers — 91

III Cholinesterase Estimations — 92

IV Centres Holding Supplies of Pralidoxime — P2S — 99

Introduction

1. This booklet is designed to help you if you are called to see a patient believed to have been poisoned by a pesticide.

2. The number of chemicals used for the control of pests, diseases and weeds in agriculture, horticulture, food storage etc continues to increase. Most of them present little or no danger to man but some are poisonous and a few intensely so. This booklet is concerned with the toxic effects that may arise through misuse or accident to agricultural workers and others handling pesticides. It does not deal with pesticide residues in food as such residues do not present a hazard to the consumer when pesticides are used in accordance with the official recommendations.

3. Before pesticides are offered for sale in the United Kingdom precise conditions of use designed to avoid any hazard to man, livestock, domestic animals and wild life are formally agreed under the Pesticides Safety Precautions Scheme. These conditions are then embodied in officially published recommendations and are also displayed on the package and container labels or associated leaflets supplied to users. Provided the directions for use are carefully followed no harm is likely to arise but people may be excessively exposed and accidents may occur when label or leaflet instructions are disregarded. Whilst exposure in itself does not mean that toxic symptoms will invariably follow, medical advice on the possible consequences and treatment is frequently sought. In practice, the more serious cases of pesticide misadventure occur from deliberate self-poisoning.

4. As many pesticide chemicals fall into distinct toxicological groups, the signs, symptoms and treatment are described in these notes under a series of collective headings with the more commonly used examples of each class referred to by their 'common' or chemical names. These should always appear on the labels of all products on the market. It may happen, nevertheless, that the doctor is informed only of a proprietary name and thus may not know the active components. An Index, listing many of the active ingredients and Trade Names of pesticide formulations commercially

available, together with their appropriate toxicological class, is therefore included in this booklet (see pages 5 to 31). Further information and advice can be obtained by telephoning one of the National Poisons Information Centres (see page i) at any hour of the day or night. In any case of alleged or suspected poisoning it is most important that the full name appearing on the label is noted. It should also be borne in mind that the clinical picture may be complicated by the effects of any organic solvents in which the pesticide principals may be dissolved.

5. When symptoms develop after exposure to a pesticide a causal association does not necessarily exist between the two events. Whilst a diagnosis of pesticide poisoning should obviously be considered and evaluated the possibility of an unrelated disease or disorder existing fortuitously should always be borne in mind.

6. Certain agricultural and horticultural chemicals which are regarded as of the highest potential danger to users are 'scheduled' under the Health and Safety (Agriculture) (Poisonous Substances) Regulations (see Appendix I) and handling conditions of such chemicals are statutorily enforced by the staff of the Health and Safety Executive's Agricultural Inspectorate. The presence of scheduled chemicals must be indicated on the product labels. The names of the chemicals specified in this way appear in the notes which follow.

7. In order that appropriate action can be taken to prevent further cases of poisoning, the circumstances leading to each pesticide incident occurring in agriculture, horticulture and forestry are investigated. Technical aspects are examined by Agricultural Inspectors and medical aspects by Employment Medical Advisers of the Health and Safety Executive. Addresses and telephone numbers of Senior Employment Medical Advisers are listed in Appendix II. When appropriate, incidents may also be appraised by the Agricultural Poisoning Appraisal Panel (APAP): such information is strictly confidential to medical staff of the Government Departments involved. Physicians may find it helpful to enlist the advice of the local Employment Medical Adviser, subject to the patient's consent, and should, in any case, inform the appropriate Poisons Information Centre of all cases of pesticide poisoning.

8. In the compilation of this booklet the help is gratefully acknowledged of medical officers and scientists in Government Departments and the pesticide industry as well as various independent experts. The text has been approved by the Advisory Committee on Pesticides, the Agricultural Departments, the Health and Safety Executive, the Directors of the National Poisons Information Services and the Health Departments.

Primary Treatment Measures

These notes are intended to summarise the first aid treatment necessary for poisoning by pesticides, with any additional special measures necessary in cases of poisoning by the more toxic pesticides.

When a person who has been using pesticides becomes ill, appropriate first aid measures should be applied and the patient sent to hospital as quickly as possible.

Always remove the patient from the spraying area into shelter if possible.

Keep the patient at rest.

Remove all protective clothing and any other clothing which may be wet with chemical, taking care to avoid contamination yourself. Wash contaminated skin thoroughly with soap and cold water.

If breathing ceases or weakens: start artificial respiration immediately, making sure the airway is clear.

If the patient has swallowed a pesticide and is conscious, vomiting should be induced by the administration of ipecacuanha (10-30 ml Ipecacuanha Emetic Mixture, Paediatric, BP) followed by 200 ml water. If there is no response a similar dose can be given after 20 minutes. Pharyngeal stimulation is not always reliable, whilst the administration of salt solution is now definitely contraindicated. Gastric lavage, taking care to prevent aspiration of fluid into the lungs, can also be used to empty the stomach but, unless carried out within four hours, it should not be considered except for the most toxic and rapidly acting substances. Induction of vomiting and washout is contraindicated following ingestion of corrosives and hydrocarbon solvents.

If contaminated with pesticide the eye should be copiously irrigated with clean water for at least 15 minutes with the eyelids held open and then covered with a soft pad of sterilized cotton wool kept firmly in position by a shade or bandage.

When the patient is being transported to hospital it is important to ensure that breathing is maintained, the airway is kept clear and the inhalation of vomit prevented. It is of the utmost importance to inform the hospital of the name of the chemical or preparation the patient has been using and to make available any label (or a copy of the label) and other information on the container together with any accompanying product leaflets.

Additional Special Measures

Arsenic Poisoning. If the patient has swallowed a chemical containing arsenic, induce vomiting and give liquids by mouth, eg milk or water.

Organochlorine Poisoning. If the patient is in a convulsion, loosen all clothing and prevent injury by gentle restraint. Intravenous diazepam should be given as soon as possible by slow injection.

Dinitro Poisoning. It is particularly important to keep the patient lying flat and at absolute rest. On no account permit him to walk or undertake any other physical exercise. Every effort should be made to keep him cool by ensuring that he is in the shade and in a free current of air, produced if necessary by fanning. All unnecessary clothing should be removed and the face and body sponged with cold water freely and frequently. If he is able to swallow, induce him to drink as much water or sweet tea as possible.

Organophosphorous and Insecticidal Carbamate Poisoning. Watch the patient's respiration carefully as it may stop suddenly. Remove false teeth in case convulsions supervene and make sure the airway is clear. Artificial respiration should be started at the first sign of respiratory failure and continued for as long as necessary. The patient should be kept at absolute rest.

Index to Diagnosis and Treatment Section by active ingredients and trade names

This index lists many of the active ingredients and Trade Names of pesticide formulations commercially available. Capital letters in the first column refer to Trade Names and small case letters to active ingredients. Each Trade Name has its principal active ingredients listed to its right. The numbers in the right-hand column refer to the relevant pesticide group described in the Diagnosis and Treatment section of this Booklet. **The abbreviation 'misc'** refers to those active ingredients or Trade Names for which the toxicological effects preclude assignment to these groups. Where such active ingredients are implicated in cases of poisoning, treatment should be directed to symptomatic and supportive measures, **including any relevant primary treatment measures described at page 3.**

Alphabetical list of trade names or active ingredients	Active Ingredient(s)	Relevant Diagnosis and Treatment Section
AAPROTECT	ziram	15
AATERRA	etridiazole	Misc.
ABOL DERRIS DUST	rotenone	Misc.
ABOL-X	gamma-HCH + menazon	3 + 4
Acephate		4
Acifluorfen		Misc.
ACREX	dinobuton	1
ACTELLIC	pirimiphos-methyl	4
ACTELLIFOG	pirimiphos-methyl	4
ACTRIL C	ioxynil + mecoprop	2 + 12
ACTRILAWN	ioxynil	2
ACUMEN	bentazone + MCPA + MCPB	12
AFALON	linuron	Misc.
AFUGAN	pyrazophos	4
AGRITOX	MCPA	12
AGROSAN D	(organomercury compound)	7
AGROTHION	fenitrothion	4

Alphabetical list of trade names or active ingredients	Active Ingredient(s)	Relevant Diagnosis and Treatment Section
AGROXONE M	MCPA	12
Alachlor		Misc.
ALANAP	naptalam	Misc.
ALAR	daminozide	Misc.
ALDERSTAN EC30	aldrin	3
Aldicarb		5
ALDREX 30	aldrin	3
ALDRIN	aldrin	3
Aldrin		3
ALGINEX	quinonamid	3
ALIBI	bifenox + linuron	Misc.
ALICEP	chloridazon + chlorbufam	Misc.
ALIETTE	aluminium ethylphosphite	Misc.
Allethrin		10
ALLISAN	dicloran	Misc.
Alloxydim-sodium		Misc.
Alphachloralose		3
Alpha-chlorohydrin		Misc.
Aluminium ethylphosphite		Misc.
AMBUSH	permethrin	10
AMCIDE	ammonium sulphamate	Misc.
Ametryne		16
AMIBEN	chloramben	12
Aminotriazole		Misc.
Amiton		4
Amitraz		Misc.
AMITROLE	aminotriazole	12
Ammonium sulphamate		Misc.
Ancymidol		Misc.
ANIMERT	tetrasul	Misc.
ANTHIO	formothion	4
Anthraquinone		Misc.
ANTI-ANT DUSTER	pyrethrum	10
ANTI-ANT POWDER	pyrethrum	10
ANTOR	diethatyl	Misc.
ANTRACOL	propineb	15
APHOX	pirimicarb	5
ARELON LIQUID	isoproturon	Misc.
ARESIN	monolinuron	Misc.
ARKOTINE-DDT	DDT	3
ARMILLATOX	cresylic acid	Misc.

Alphabetical list of trade names or active ingredients	Active Ingredient(s)	Relevant Diagnosis and Treatment Section
AROTEX SC	chlormequat	Misc.
ARRESIN	monolinuron	Misc.
ARREST-A-PEST RAT BAIT	warfarin	18
Arsenious oxide		9
Asulam		Misc.
ASULOX	asulam	Misc.
ATLACIDE EXTRA DUSTING POWDER	sodium chlorate + atrazine	16 + 17
ATLACIDE SOLUBLE POWDER	sodium chlorate	17
ATLADOX HI	picloram	12
ATLASETOX	demephion	4
ATLAVER	sodium chlorate + atrazine + 2,4-D	12 + 16 + 17
ATLAZIN	aminotriazole + atrazine	12 + 16
Atrazine		16
AUTUMN TOPLAWN	carbaryl + quintozene	5
AVADEX	di-allate	Misc.
AVADEX BW	tri-allate	Misc.
AVENGE	difenzoquat	Misc.
AVENTOX SC	simazine + trietazine	16
AZATHION	azinphos-methyl	4
Azinphos-ethyl		4
Azinphos-methyl		4
Aziprotryne		16
Azocyclotin		13
AZODRIN	monocrotophos	4
AZOTOX	demeton-s-methyl	4
B25	barban	Misc.
BAN-DOCK	2,4,5-T + mecoprop + dicamba	12
BANLENE PLUS	dicamba + mecoprop + MCPA	12
BANVEL	dicamba	12
Barban		Misc.
BARDEW	tridemorph	Misc.
BASAGRAN	bentazone	Misc.
BASAMID	dazomet	Misc.
BASUDIN	diazinon	4
BAVISTIN	carbendazim	Misc.
BAYGON	propoxur	5
BAYLETON	triadimefon	Misc.
BAYTHION	phoxim	4

BEN

Alphabetical list of trade names or active ingredients	Active Ingredient(s)	Relevant Diagnosis and Treatment Section
BENAZALOX	3,6-dichloropicolinic acid + benazolin	12
Benazolin		12
Bendiocarb		5
BENLATE	benomyl	Misc.
BENLATE T	benomyl + thiram	Misc. + 15
Benomyl		Misc.
Bentazone		Misc.
Benthiocarb		Misc.
BENTROL	bromoxynil	2
Benzoylprop-ethyl		Misc.
BERELEX	gibberellic acid	Misc.
BETANAL E	phenmedipham	Misc.
BH43	maleic hydrazide + 2,4-D	12
BIDISIN	chlorfenprop-methyl	4
Bifenox		Misc.
Binapacryl		1
Bioallethrin		10
BIO BACK TO NATURE INSECT SPRAY	rotenone + quassia	Misc.
BIO BACK TO NATURE PEST & DISEASE DUSTER	rotenone	Misc.
BIO LAWN WEEDKILLER	ioxynil + 2,4-D + dicamba	2 + 12
BIO MOSS KILLER	dichlorophen	Misc.
Bioresmethrin		10
BIO SPRAYDAY	pyrethrum + resmethrin	10
BIOSYSTEMIC INSECTICIDE	dimethoate	4
BIRLANE	chlorfenvinphos	4
BLADAFUM	sulfotep	4
BLAGAL	cyanazine + MCPA	16 + 12
BLATTANEX	propoxur	5
BLAZER	acifluorfen	Misc.
BOOTS ANT DESTROYER	gamma-HCH	3
BOOTS CALOMEL DUST	mercurous chloride	8
BOOTS DERRIS DUST	derris	Misc.
BOOTS GARDEN INSECT KILLER	gamma-HCH + pyrethrins + piperonyl butoxide	3 + 10 + Misc.
BOOTS GARDEN INSECT POWDER	carbaryl	5
BOOTS GREENFLY KILLER	malathion	4
BOOTS LAWN FERTILIZER AND WEEDKILLER	2,4-D + mecoprop	12

Alphabetical list of trade names or active ingredients	Active Ingredient(s)	Relevant Diagnosis and Treatment Section
BOOTS LAWN WEED/FEED	dichlorprop + MCPA	12
BOOTS LAWN WEEDKILLER	2,4-D + mecoprop	12
BOOTS MOSSKILLER AND FERTILIZER	ferrous sulphate	Misc.
BOOTS SLUG DESTROYER	metaldehyde	Misc.
BOOTS SODIUM CHLORATE	sodium chlorate	17
BOOTS SYSTEMIC GREENFLY KILLER	dimethoate	4
BOTRILEX	PCNB (quintozene)	Misc.
BRASORAN 50WP	aziprotryne	16
BRASSICOL	PCNB (quintozene)	Misc.
BRAVO 500	chlorothalonil	Misc.
BRESTAN 60	maneb + fentin acetate	15 + 13
BRITTOX	bromoxynil + ioxynil + mecoprop	2 + 12
Brodifacoum		18
Bromacil		Misc.
Bromadiolone		18
Bromofenoxim		1
BROMOPHOS	bromophos	4
Bromophos		4
Bromopropylate		Misc.
Bromoxynil		2
BRONOX	trietazine	16
BUCTRIL M	bromoxynil + MCPA	2 + 12
Bupirimate		Misc.
BURTOLIN	maleic hydrazide	Misc.
Butam		Misc.
BUTOXONE M	2,4-D + 2,4-DB + MCPA	12
Butoxycarboxim		5
Butylate		Misc.
CALIXIN	tridemorph	Misc.
CALOMEL DUST	mercurous chloride	8
CAMBILENE	2,3,6-TBA + mecoprop + MCPA + dicamba	12
CAMBELL'S	nabam	15
Camphechlor		3
CAMTOX	2,3,6-TBA + 2,4-DP + mecoprop	12
Captafol		Misc.
Captan		Misc.
CARBAMULT	promecarb	5

Alphabetical list of trade names or active ingredients	Active Ingredient(s)	Relevant Diagnosis and Treatment Section
Carbaryl		5
Carbendazim		Misc.
CARBETAMEX	carbetamide	Misc.
Carbetamide		Misc.
Carbofuran		5
Carbon tetrachloride		19(b)
Carbophenothion		Misc.
Carboxin		Misc.
CARBYNE	barban	Misc.
CASORAN G	dichlobenil	Misc.
CATERPILLAR KILLER (DIPTEREX)	trichlorphon	4
CERCOBIN	thiophanate methyl	15
CERESOL	mercury (organomercury fungicide)	7
CERONE	ethephon	Misc.
CERTROL PA	ioxynil + dichlorprop + MCPA	2 + 12
CERTROL-LIN ONIONS	ioxynil + linuron	2 + Misc.
CHANDOR	trifluralin + linuron	Misc.
CHILDION	dicofol + tetradifon	Misc. + 3
Chloramben		12
Chloraniformethan		Misc.
Chlorbromuron		Misc.
Chlorbufam		Misc.
CHLORDANE	chlordane	3
Chlordane		3
Chlorfenprop-methyl		Misc.
Chlorfenvinphos		4
Chloridazon		Misc.
Chlormequat		Misc.
Chlorophacinone		18
Chloropicrin		19(e)
Chlorothalonil		Misc.
Chloroxuron		Misc.
Chlorpropham		Misc.
Chlorpyrifos		4
Chlorpyrifos-methyl		4
Chlorthal-dimethyl		12
Chlorthiamid		Misc.
Chlortoluron		Misc.
CIDIAL	phenthoate	4
CIPC	chlorpropham	Misc.

Alphabetical list of trade names or active ingredients	Active Ingredient(s)	Relevant Diagnosis and Treatment Section
CLAROSAN	terbutryne	16
CLEANSWEEP	diquat + paraquat	11
CLEAVAL	cyanazine + mecoprop	16 + 12
CLOUT	alloxydim-sodium	Misc.
CLOVERCIDE EXTRA	ioxynil + mecoprop	2 + 12
CLOVOTOX	mecoprop	12
CMPP	CMPP	12
COBEX	dinitramine	Misc.
COMMANDO	flamprop-isopropyl	Misc.
Copper aceto arsenite		6
Copper oxychloride		Misc.
CORBEL	fenpropemorph	12
CORNOX 290 PLUS	3,6-dichloropicolinic acid + dichlorprop + MCPA	Misc. + 12
CORNOXYNIL	bromoxynil + 2,4-DP	2 + 12
COSMIC	carbendazim + maneb + tridemorph	15
Coumatetralyl		18
Cresylic Acid		Misc.
COUNTER 2G	terbufos	4
CRONETON	ethiofencarb	5
CROP SAVER	malathion + resmethrin + trichlorphon	4 + 10
CROTOTHANE	dinocap	1
CUFRAM Z	cufraneb	15
Cufraneb		15
CUPROKYLT	copper oxychloride	Misc.
CUTLASS	dikegulac	Misc.
Cyanazine		16
Cyanides		19(g)
Cycloate		Misc.
CYCLOSAN	mercurous chloride	8
CYCOCEL	chlormequat	Misc.
Cyhexatin		13
Cypermethrin		10
CYTHION	malathion	4
CYTRO-LANE	mephosfolan	4
2,4-D	2,4-D	12
2,4-DB	2,4-DB	12
2,4-DES	2,4-DES	12
2,4-DP	dichlorprop	12

3,6-D

Alphabetical list of trade names or active ingredients	Active Ingredient(s)	Relevant Diagnosis and Treatment Section
3,6-Dichloropicolinic Acid		Misc.
D50	2,4-D	12
DACONIL 2787	chlorothalonil	Misc.
DACTHAL	chlorthal-dimethyl	12
DALAPON	dalapon	Misc.
Dalapon		Misc.
Daminozide		Misc.
Dazomet		Misc.
DDT		3
DDVP	dichlorvos	4
Decamethrin		10
DECAMOX	thiofanox	5
DECIS	deltamethrin	10
DEFTOR	metoxuron	Misc.
DELAN-COL	dithianon	Misc.
DELNAV	dioxathion	4
DELOXIL	bromoxynil + ioxynil	2
DELOZIN S	chlorthal-dimethyl + methazole	12 + Misc.
DELSENE M	carbendazim + maneb	Misc. + 15
Deltamethrin		10
Demephion		4
Demeton		4
Demeton-methyl		4
Demeton-S-methyl		4
Demeton-S-methyl sulphone		4
DEROSAL	carbendazim	Misc.
DERRIS	rotenone	Misc.
DERRIS DUST	rotenone	Misc.
Desmetryne		16
DEVRINOL	napropamide	Misc.
DEXURON	diuron + paraquat	Misc. + 11
Di-allate		Misc.
Dialifos		4
Diazinon		4
DI-SYSTON	disulfoton	4
DI-TRAPEX	methyl isothiocyanate	Misc.
DIBROM	naled	4
Dicamba		12
DICARZOL	formetanate (as hydrochloride)	5
Dichlobenil		Misc.
Dichlofluanid		Misc.
Dichlorophen		Misc.

DIC

Alphabetical list of trade names or active ingredients	Active Ingredient(s)	Relevant Diagnosis and Treatment Section
Dichloropropane		Misc.
Dichlorprop		12
Dichlorvos		4
Diclofop-methyl		12
Dicloran		Misc.
DICOFEN	fenitrothion	4
Dicofol		3
Dicophane (DDT)	DDT	3
DICOTOX EXTRA	2,4-D	12
DICRON 45SC	phosphamidon	4
DICURAN	chlortoluron	Misc.
Dieldrin		3
Dienochlor		3
Difenacoum		18
Difenzoquat		Misc.
Diflubenzuron		Misc.
DIFOLATAN	captafol	Misc.
Dikegulac		Misc.
DIMECRON	phosphamidon	4
Dimefox		4
Dimethirimol		Misc.
Dimethoate		4
DIMILIN	diflubenzuron	Misc.
Dinitramine		Misc.
Dinitro ortho cresol		1
Dinobuton		1
Dinocap		1
Dinoseb		1
Dinoterb		1
Dioxacarb		5
Dioxathion		4
DIPHACIN 120	diphacinone	18
Diphacinone		18
Diphenamid		Misc.
Diphenyltin		13
DIPTEREX 80	trichlorfon	4
Diquat		11
Disulfoton		4
Ditalimfos		4
DITHANE 945	mancozeb	15
DITHANE A40	nabam	15
DITHANE M-22	maneb	15

13

Alphabetical list of trade names or active ingredients	Active Ingredient(s)	Relevant Diagnosis and Treatment Section
DITHANE M-45	mancozeb	15
DITHANE WETTABLE	zineb	15
DITHANE Z-78	zineb	15
Dithianon		Misc.
Diuron		Misc.
DNOC	DNOC	1
DNBP	dinoseb	1
Dodemorph		Misc.
Dodine		Misc.
DORMONE	2,4-D	12
DOSAFLOR	metoxuron	Misc.
DOSANEX	metoxuron	Misc.
DOUBLEDOWN	disulfoton + fonofos	4
DOUBLET	bromoxynil + ioxynil + isoproturon	2 + Misc.
DOWFUME	methyl bromide	19(a)
DOWPON	dalapon	Misc.
DRAT	chlorophacinone	18
DRAZA	mercaptodimethur	5
DRAZA SLUG PELLETS	methiocarb	5
Drazoxolon		Misc.
DU-TER	fentin hydroxide	13
DUAL	metolachlor	Misc.
DURSBAN	chlorpyrifos	4
DYFONATE	fonofos	4
ECONAL	2,4,5-T	12
EKAMET	etrimfos	4
EKATIN	thiometon	4
ELECRON	dioxacarb	5
ELOCRIL 50WP	iodofenphos	4
ELOSAL	sulphur	Misc.
ELVARON	dichlofluanid	Misc.
EMBARK	mefluidide	Misc.
EMBUTOX	2,4-DB	12
EMBUTOX PLUS	2,4-D + MCPA	12
Endosulfan		3
Endrin		3
ENIDE 50W	diphenamid	Misc.
EPIBLOC	alpha-chlorohydrin	Misc.
EPTAM	EPTC	Misc.
EPTC	EPTC	Misc.

Alphabetical list of trade names or active ingredients	Active Ingredient(s)	Relevant Diagnosis and Treatment Section
ERADICANE	EPTC + protectant	Misc.
Ethephon		Misc.
Ethiofencarb		5
Ethion		4
Ethirimol		Misc.
Ethoate-methyl		4
Ethofumesate		Misc.
Ethoprophos		4
Ethoxyquin		Misc.
ETHREL	ethephon	Misc.
Ethyl mercury phosphate		7
Ethylene dibromide		19(d)
Ethylene dichloride		19(c)
Etridiazole		Misc.
Etrimfos		4
EUPAREN	dichlofluanid	Misc.
EUPAREN M	tolyfluanid	Misc.
EVERGREEN 80	2,4-D + dicamba	12
EVERGREEN FOAMING SPOT WEEDKILLER	2,4-D + dicamba	12
EVERGREEN LAWN WEEDKILLER	2,4-D + dicamba	12
EVIK 80W	ametryne	16
F 238	dodemorph	Misc.
FAC 20	prothoate	4
FANERON COMBI	terbuthylazine + bromofenoxim	16 + 1
FARMIL	ditalimfos	4
FARMON 2,4-DB PLUS	2,4-DB + MCPA	12
FARMON CONDOX M	dicamba + mecoprop	12
Fenarimol		Misc.
Fenbutatin oxide		13
Fenchlorphos		4
FENITROTHION	fenitrothion	4
Fenitrothion		4
Fenoprop		Misc.
Fenpropemorph		12
Fenthion		4
Fentin acetate		13
Fentin hydroxide		13
Fenuron		Misc.
Fenvalerate		Misc.

FER

Alphabetical list of trade names or active ingredients	Active Ingredient(s)	Relevant Diagnosis and Treatment Section
Ferbam		15
FERNIMINE M	2,4-D	12
Ferrous Sulphate		Misc.
FERVIN	alloxydim-sodium	Misc.
FICAM W	bendiocarb	5
FISONS COMBAT GREEN INSECTICIDE	malathion + gamma-HCH	4
FISONS COMBAT PATH WEEDKILLER	aminotriazole + MCPA + simazine	Misc. + 12 + 16
FISONS COMBAT ROSE FUNGICIDE	carbendazim + maneb	Misc. + 15
FISONS COMBAT SLUG PELLETS	metaldehyde	Misc.
FISONS COMBAT SOIL INSECTICIDE	diazinon	4
FISONS COMBAT VEGETABLE INSECTICIDE	bioresmethrin + malathion	10 + 4
FISONS COMBAT WHITEFLY INSECTICIDE	bioresmethrin	10
FISONS LAWN SAND	ferrous sulphate	Misc.
FISONS MOSSKIL	ferrous sulphate	Misc.
Flamprop-isopropyl		Misc.
Flamprop-methyl		Misc.
Fluoracetamide		6
Fluoracetates		6
FOLIMAT	omethoate	4
Folpet		Misc.
FONGARID 25WP	furalaxyl	Misc.
Fonofos		4
FORMAT	3,6-dichloropicolinic acid	12
Formetanate		5
Formothion		4
FORTROL	cyanazine	16
Fosamine		Misc.
FOSFERNO	parathion	4
FUBOL 58 WP	mancozeb + metalaxyl	15 + Misc.
FUMITE BHC SMOKE CONE	gamma-HCH	3
FUMITE TECNALIN CONES	gamma-HCH	3
FUNGAFLOR	imazalil	Misc.
FURADAN	carbofuran	5
Furalaxyl		Misc.
FYTOSPORE	cymoxanil	Misc.

Alphabetical list of trade names or active ingredients	Active Ingredient(s)	Relevant Diagnosis and Treatment Section
Gamma-HCH		3
GAMMA-COL	gamma-HCH	3
GARDONA	tetrachlorvinphos	4
GARVOX 3G	bendiocarb	5
GESAGARD 50 WP	prometryne	16
GESAPRIM 500L	atrazine	16
GESARAN 2079	methoprotryne + simazine	16
GESATOP 500L	simazine	16
Gibberillic acid		Misc.
Glyphosate		Misc.
GOLTIX	metamitron	Misc.
GRAMONOL	monolinuron	Misc.
GRAMOXONE	paraquat	11
GRASLAM	asulam	Misc.
Guazatine		Misc.
GULF BUTAM	butam	Misc.
GUSATHION MS	azinphos-methyl	4
HAULMEX	dinoseb in oil	1
HCH	gamma-HCH	3
Heptenophos		4
HERALD	chloridazon + fenuron + propham + chlorpropham	Misc.
HERBITOX	dicamba + dichlorprop + benazolin	12
HERBON 2,4-DES	2,4-DES	12
HERBON BLUE	2,4-DES + simazine	12 + 16
HERBON BROWN	pentanochlor + chlorpropham	Misc.
HERBON DALAPON	dalapon	Misc.
HERBON GARDEN HERBICIDE	CIPC + diuron + IPC	Misc.
HERBON GOLD	propham + fenuron + chlorpropham	Misc.
HERBON ORANGE	propachlor	Misc.
HERBON SOLAN 40	pentanochlor	Misc.
HERBON SOMON	sodium chlorate	17
HERRISOL PLUS	2,3,6-TBA + mecoprop + MCPA + dicamba	12
Hexazinone		Misc.
HEXYL	gamma-HCH + rotenone + thiram	Misc. + 15
HOEGRASS	diclofop-methyl	12
HOSTAQUICK	heptenophos	4

Alphabetical list of trade names or active ingredients	Active Ingredient(s)	Relevant Diagnosis and Treatment Section
HOSTATHION	triazophos	4
HOUSE/GARDEN PLANT PEST KILLER	pyrethrum + resmethrin	10
HURSTMASTER	dalapon + MCPA	12 + Misc.
HYDON	picloram	12
Hydrogen cyanide		19(g)
HYMEC	mecoprop	12
HYQUAT	chlormequat	Misc.
HYSWARD	mecoprop + MCPA + dicamba	12
HYTANE 500L	isoproturon	Misc.
HYVAR X	bromacil	Misc.
4-Indol-3-ylbutyric acid		Misc.
ICI ANTKILLER	pirimiphos-methyl	4
ICI CLUB ROOT CONTROL	mercurous chloride	8
ICI GENERAL GARDEN FUNGICIDE	thiram	Misc.
ICI MOSSKILLER FOR LAWNS	ferrous sulphate	Misc.
ICI SLUG PELLETS	metaldehyde	Misc.
ICI SODIUM CHLORATE WITH FIRE DEPRESSANT	sodium chlorate	17
IGRAN	terbutryne	16
Imazalil		Misc.
IMIDAN	phosmet	4
Iodofenphos		4
IOTOX	ioxynil + mecoprop	2 + 12
Ioxynil		2
Iprodione		Misc.
Iron chelate		Misc.
Isoproturon		Misc.
IVORIN	monolinuron + dinoseb acetate	Misc. + 1
IVOSIT	dinoseb acetate	1
KARATHANE	dinocap	1
Karbutilate		Misc.
KARMEX	diuron	Misc.
KELTHANE 20	dicofol	3
KERB 50W	propyzamide	Misc.
KERISPRAY	pirimiphos-methyl	4
KEYTROL	2,4-D + aminotriazole + atrazine	12 + 16 + Misc.
KILNET	2,4-D + 2,4,5-T	12

KIL

Alphabetical list of trade names or active ingredients	Active Ingredient(s)	Relevant Diagnosis and Treatment Section
KILVAL	vamidothion	4
KLOBEN	neburon	Misc.
KOMBAT	carbendazim + mancozeb	Misc. + 15
KORLAN	fenchlorphos	4
KRENITE	fosamine	Misc.
KROVAR 1	bromacil + diuron	Misc.
KUMULAN	nitrothal-isopropyl + sulphur	Misc.
LANCER	flamprop-methyl	Misc.
LANDSLIDE	linuron + lenacil	Misc.
LANNATE	methomyl	5
LASSO	alachlor	Misc.
LAWN 'PLUS'	2,4-D + dicamba	12
Lead arsenate		9
LEBAYCID	fenthion	4
LEGUMEX EXTRA	2,4-DB + MCPA + benazolin	12
Lenacil		Misc.
LEY-CORNOX	2,4-DB + benazolin + MCPA	12
LEY-HERBITOX	2,4-DB + benazolin + MCPA	12
LIGNASAN	carbendazim	Misc.
LINDANE	gamma-HCH	3
LINNET	linuron + trifluralin	Misc.
Linuron		Misc.
LIQUID DERRIS	rotenone	Misc.
LONTREL	3,6-dichloropicolinic acid + 2,4-DP	Misc. + 12
LONTREL PLUS	3,6-dichloropicolinic acid + 2,4-DP + MCPA	Misc. + 12
M & B SOIL INSECTICIDE GRANULES	diazinon	4
M-C	mercurous chloride	8
M36	MCPA	12
Malathion		4
MALATHION GREENFLY KILLER	malathion	4
Maleic hydrazide		Misc.
MALET 50EC	ioxynil + mecoprop	2 + 12
MALORAN 50 WP	chlorbromuron	Misc.
MAMBAR	chlormequat	Misc.
Mancozeb		15
Maneb		15

19

MAN

Alphabetical list of trade names or active ingredients	Active Ingredient(s)	Relevant Diagnosis and Treatment Section
Manganese and zinc dithiocarbamate		15
MARLATE	methoxychlor	3
MATRIKERB	3,6-dichloropicolinic acid + propyzamide	12 + Misc.
MAZIDE	maleic hydrazide	Misc.
Mazidox		4
MAZIN	maneb + zinc oxide	15
MCPA	MCPA	12
MCPB	MCPB	12
Mecarbam		4
Mecoprop		12
Medinoterb		1
Mefluidide		Misc.
MELPREX	dodine	Misc.
Menazon		4
Mephosfolan		4
Mepiquat chloride		11
Mercaptodimethur = (methiocarb)		5
Mercuric oxide		8
Mercurous Chloride		8
Mercury (organomercury fungicide)		7
MERGAMMA	gamma HCH + organomercury compound	3 + 7
MESUROL	mercaptodimethur	5
Metalaxyl		Misc.
Metaldehyde		Misc.
Metamitron		Misc.
METASYSTOX 55	demeton-s-methyl	4
METASYSTOX R	oxydemeton-methyl	4
Methabenzthiazuron		Misc.
Metham sodium		15
Methamidophos		4
Methazole		Misc.
Methidathion		4
Methiocarb		5
Methomyl		5
Methoprotryne		16
METHOXONE M	mecoprop	12
Methoxychlor		3
Methoxyethyl mercury acetate		7

MET

Alphabetical list of trade names or active ingredients	Active Ingredient(s)	Relevant Diagnosis and Treatment Section
Methoxyethyl mercury chloride		7
Methyl bromide		19
Methyl isothiocyanate		Misc.
Metiram		15
Metobromuron		Misc.
Metolachlor		Misc.
Metoxuron		Misc.
Metribuzin		Misc.
Mevinphos		4
MIDOX FORTE	aminotriazole + simazine + MCPA	Misc. + 12 + 16
MIL-COL 30	drazoxolon	Misc.
MILCAP	captafol + ethirimol	Misc.
MILCURB	dimethirimol	Misc.
MILDOTHANE	thiophanate-methyl	Misc.
MILFARON	chloraniformethan	Misc.
MILGO-E	ethirimol	Misc.
MILSTEM	ethirimol	Misc.
MISTRAL	fenpropemorph	12
MITAC 20	amitraz	Misc.
MOCAP	ethoprophos	4
MODOWN	bifenox	Misc.
MOFIX 50 EC	bromofenoxin	1
Molinate		Misc.
MOFIX 500L	terbuthylazine + bromofenoxim	16 + 1
MONITOR	methamidophos	4
Monocrotophos		4
Monolinuron		Misc.
MORESTAN	quinomethionate	Misc.
MORKIT	anthraquinone	Misc.
MORLEX	ethofumesate + chlorpropham + propham + fenuron	Misc.
MOROCIDE	binapacryl	1
MOS-TOX	mercurous chloride	8
MOSSTOX PLUS	dichlorophen	Misc.
MURBENINE	guazatine	Misc.
MURFOTOX	mecarbam	4
MURFOTOX OIL	mecarbam	4
MURFUME BHC SMOKE CONE	gamma-HCH	3
MURFUME DINOCAP SMOKE (CONE)	dinocap	1

MUR

Alphabetical list of trade names or active ingredients	Active Ingredient(s)	Relevant Diagnosis and Treatment Section
MURFUME LINDANE SMOKE PELLETS	gamma-HCH	3
MURFUME PARATHION SMOKE	parathion	4
MURGANIC RPB	carboxin	Misc.
MURPHY CALOMEL DUST	mercurous chloride	8
MURPHY CHLORDANE WORMKILLER	chlordane	3
MURPHY COMBINED PEST & DISEASE DUST	rotenone + sulphur + zineb	Misc. + 15
MURPHY COMBINED PEST & DISEASE SPRAY	dicofol + dinocap + fenitrothion + maneb + pyrethrum	3 + 1 + 4 + 15 + 10
MURPHY COMBINED SEED DRESSING	captan + gamma-HCH	Misc.
MURPHY DERRIS DUST	rotenone	Misc.
MURPHY DERRIS LIQUID	rotenone	Misc.
MURPHY DINOCAP MILDEW FUNGICIDE	dinocap	1
MURPHY FENTRO	fenitrothion	4
MURPHY GAMMA-BHC DUST	gamma-HCH	3
MURPHY GREENHOUSE AEROSOL	malathion	4
MURPHY LAWN FOOD PLUS WEED CONTROL	2,4-D + fenoprop + mecoprop	12 + Misc.
MURPHY LAWN WEEDKILLER	2,4-D + dichlorprop	12
MURPHY LINDEX GARDEN SPRAY	gamma-HCH	3
MURPHY LIQUID MALATHION	malathion	4
MURPHY MALATHION DUST	malathion	4
MURPHY ORTHOCIDE CAPTAN FUNGICIDE	captan	Misc.
MURPHY ROSE FUNGICIDE	dinocap + folpet	1 + Misc.
MURPHY SEVIN DUST	carbaryl	5
MURPHY SLUGIT LIQUID	metaldehyde	Misc.
MURPHY SODIUM CHLORATE	sodium chlorate	17
MURPHY SOIL PEST KILLER	chlorpyrifos	4

Alphabetical list of trade names or active ingredients	Active Ingredient(s)	Relevant Diagnosis and Treatment Section
MURPHY SUPER MOSS-KILLER & LAWN FUNGICIDE	dichlorophen	Misc.
MURPHY SYSTEMIC CLUB ROOT DIP	thiophanate-methyl	Misc.
MURPHY SYSTEMIC FUNGICIDE	thiophanate-methyl	Misc.
MURPHY SYSTEMIC INSECTICIDE	dimethoate	4
MURPHY TUMBLEBUG	heptenophos + permethrin	4 + 10
MURPHY TUMBLEWEED	glyphosate	Misc.
MURPHY WASP DESTROYER	carbaryl	5
MURVIN 85	carbaryl	5
NAA		Misc.
Nabam		15
Naled		4
Napropamide		Misc.
Naptalam		Misc.
NATA	TCA	Misc.
Neburon		Misc.
NEMAFOS	thionazin	4
NEO-PYNAMIN	tetramethrin	10
NEORON	bromopropylate	Misc.
NEOSOREXA	difenacoum	18
NETTLE-BAN	2,4,5-T + 2,4-D + dicamba	12
NEW CLOVOTOX	ioxynil + mecoprop	2 + 12
NEXION	bromophos	4
Nicotine		14
NIMROD	bupirimate	Misc.
NIMROD-T	bupirimate + triforine	Misc.
NIPPON AEROSOL SPRAY	chlordane + piperonyl butoxide + pyrethrins	3 + 10
NIPPON ANT POWDER	chlordane	3
NIPPON ANT, WASP & CRAWLING INSECT SPRAY	chlordane	3
Nitrofen		Misc.
Nitrothal-isopropyl		Misc.
NOGOS 50EC	dichlorvos	4
NORTRON	ethofumesate	Misc.

Alphabetical list of trade names or active ingredients	Active Ingredient(s)	Relevant Diagnosis and Treatment Section
Omethoate		4
OMITE	propargite	Misc.
OPOGARD 500L	terbuthylazine + terbutryne	16
ORDRAM	molinate	Misc.
ORTHENE	acephate	4
ORTHO DIFOLATAN	captafol	Misc.
ORTHO PHALTAN	folpet	Misc.
ORTHOCIDE	captan	Misc.
Oxadiazon		Misc.
Oxamyl		5
Oxycarboxin		Misc.
Oxydemeton-methyl		4
OXYTRIL P	bromoxynil + ioxynil + dichlorprop	2 + 12
PALLINAL	nitrothal-isopropyl with zineb-polyethylene thiram disulphide complex	Misc. + 15
PANAGEN M	organomercury compound	7
Paraquat		11
Parathion		4
PATHCLEAR	paraquat + diquat + simazine	11 + 16
PATORAN	metobromuron	Misc.
PCNB		Misc.
Pendimethalin		Misc.
PENTAC	dienochlor	3
Pentachlorophenol		2
Pentanochlor		Misc.
Permethrin		10
PERMIT	permethrin	10
PEROPAL	azocyclotin	13
PERSELECT	2,4-DB + MCPA	12
PESTAN	mecarbam	4
Phenkapton		4
Phenmedipham		12
Phenothrin		10
PHENOXYLENE SUPER	dicamba + MCPA	12
Phenthoate		4
Phenylmercury acetate		7
Phenylmercury catechol		7
Phorate		4
PHORTOX SCRUB/ NETTLE KILLER	2,4,5-T	12

PHO

Alphabetical list of trade names or active ingredients	Active Ingredient(s)	Relevant Diagnosis and Treatment Section
Phosalone		4
PHOSDRIN	mevinphos	4
Phosmet		4
Phosphamidon		4
Phosphine		19(f)
Phoxim		4
PICKET	permethrin	10
Picloram		12
Piperonyl butoxide		Misc.
Pirimicarb		5
Pirimiphos-ethyl		4
Pirimiphos-methyl		4
PIRIMOR	pirimicarb	5
PLANOTOX	2,4-D	12
PLANT PEST KILLER	pyrethrum	10
PLANT PIN	butoxycarboxim	5
PLANTINEB 80	maneb	15
PLANTVAX	oxycarboxin	Misc.
PLANTVAX 75	oxycarboxin	Misc.
PLICTRAN 25W	cyhexatin	13
PLICTRAN 600F	cyhexatin	13
PLONDREL 50W	ditalimfos	4
POLYMONE X	2,4-DP + 2,4-D	12
POLYRAM-COMBI	metiram	15
PRADONE PLUS	dimefuron + carbetamide	Misc.
PREBANE 500L	terbutryne	16
PREFIX	chlorthiamid	Misc.
PREMALOX	chlorpropham + fenuron + propham	Misc.
PREVICUR	prothiocarb	15
PRIMATOL AD 85 WP	2,4-D + atrazine + aminotriazole	12 + 16 + Misc.
PRIMATOL SE 500L	aminotriazole + simazine	Misc.
PROBE	methazole	Misc.
Prochloraz		Misc.
Procymidone		Misc.
PROFALON	chlorpropham + linuron	Misc.
Promecarb		5
Prometryne		16
Propachlor		Misc.
Propanil		Misc.
Propargite		Misc.

25

PRO

Alphabetical list of trade names or active ingredients	Active Ingredient(s)	Relevant Diagnosis and Treatment Section
PROPCORN	propionic acid	Misc.
Propham		Misc.
Propineb		15
Propionic acid		Misc.
PROPONEX-PLUS	mecoprop	12
Propoxur		5
Propyzamide		Misc.
Prothiocarb		15
Prothoate		4
PYRACIDE	demephion	4
PYRAMIN	chloridazon	Misc.
Pyrazophos		4
Pyrethrum		10
Quinalphos		4
Quinomethionate		Misc.
QUINTEX	propham + fenuron + chlorpropham	Misc.
Quintozene		Misc.
RACUMIN MOUSE BAIT	coumatetralyl	18
RACUMIN RAT BAIT	coumatetralyl	18
RAMIK	diphacinone	18
RAMROD	propachlor	Misc.
RAPID GREENFLY KILLER	pirimicarb	5
RATAK	difenacoum	18
REDUCYMOL	ancymidol	Misc.
REGLONE	diquat	11
REGULOX 50W	maleic hydrazide	Misc.
RELDAN	chlorpyrifos-methyl	4
RESIDOX	atrazine	16
RESIDUREN EXTRA	chlorpropham + diuron	Misc.
Resmethrin		10
RIPCORD	cypermethrin	10
RO-NEET	cycloate	Misc.
ROGOR	dimethoate	4
RONILAN	vinclozolin	Misc.
RONSTAR	oxadiazon	Misc.
ROOT GUARD	diazinon	4
ROSE & FLOWER PEST & DISEASE DUSTER	rotenone + carbaryl	Misc. + 5
rotenone		Misc.

Alphabetical list of trade names or active ingredients	Active Ingredient(s)	Relevant Diagnosis and Treatment Section
ROUNDUP	glyphosate	Misc.
ROVRAL	iprodione	Misc.
RUBIGAN	fenarimol	Misc.
SALVO	dazomet	Misc.
SANDOLIN A	DNOC	1
SANSPOR	captafol	Misc.
SANTAR	mercuric oxide	8
SAPECRON	chlorfenvinphos	4
SAPROL	triforine	Misc.
SATURN	benthiocarb	Misc.
SAVALL	quinalphos	4
S-Bioallethrin	quinalphos	10
SBK BRUSHWOOD KILLER	2,4-D + 2,4,5-T	12
Schradan		4
SCOTLENE	dicamba + mecoprop + MCPA	12
SEL-OXONE	3,6-dichloropicolinic acid + mecoprop	12
4-50 SELECTIVE WEEDKILLER	2,4-D + fenoprop	12 + Misc.
SEMERON 25 WP	desmetryne	16
SENCOR	metribuzin	Misc.
SENCOREX	metribuzin	Misc.
SEQUESTRENE 138 FE	iron chelate	Misc.
SERADIX	4-indol-3-ylbutyric acid	Misc.
SEVIN 85WP	carbaryl	5
SHELL D-50	2,4-D	12
SIMADEX SC	simazine	16
Simazine		16
SINBAR	terbacil	12
SISTAN	metham sodium	15
SLAYMOR	bromadiolone	18
SLUG DEATH POWDER & PELLETS	metaldehyde	Misc.
SLUG GARD	methiocarb	5
SLUG MINI PELLETS	metaldehyde	Misc.
Sodium arsenite		9
Sodium borate		Misc.
Sodium chlorate		17
Sodium monochloracetate		Misc.
SOLUBOR	sodium borate	Misc.
SOLVIGRAN	disulfoton	4

Alphabetical list of trade names or active ingredients	Active Ingredient(s)	Relevant Diagnosis and Treatment Section
SPECTRON	ethofumesate + chloridazon	Misc.
SPONTOX	2,4,5-T + 2,4-D	12
SPORTAK	prochloraz	Misc.
SPRINGCLENE	bromoxynil + ioxynil + linuron + mecoprop	2 + Misc. + 12
STAY-KLEEN	cyanazine + linuron	16 + Misc.
STEMPOR	carbendazim	Misc.
STOMP	pendimethalin	Misc.
STOP-SCALD	ethoxyquin	Misc.
STORITE	thiabendazole	Misc.
SUFFIX	benzoylprop ethyl	Misc.
Sulfallate		15
Sulfotep		4
Sulphur		Misc.
SUMICIDIN	fenvalerate	Misc.
SUMISCLEX	procymidone	Misc.
SUMITHION	fenitrothion	4
SUPER WEEDEX	aminotriazole + simazine	Misc.
SUPERLEC	maleic hydrazide	Misc.
SUPERTOX	2,4-D + mecoprop	12
SUPERTOX 30	2,4-D + mecoprop	12
SUPRACIDE 40EC	methidathion	4
SUTAN	butylate	Misc.
SYBOL 2	pirimiphos-methyl	4
SYBOL 2 AEROSOL	pirimiphos-methyl	4
SYBOL 2 DUST	pirimiphos-methyl	4
SYNCHEMICALS CALOMEL DUST	mercurous chloride	8
SYNDANE 25	chlordane	3
SYSTOX	demeton	4
2,3,6-TBA	T,3,6-TBA	12
2,4,5-T	2,4,5-T	12
TAKTIC	amitraz	Misc.
TAMARON	methamidophos	4
TANDEX	karbutilate	Misc.
TECANE	TCA	Misc.
TEDION V-18	tetradifon	Misc.
TEPP	TEPP	4
TELONE II	dichloropropane	Misc.
TEMIK	aldicarb	5
TENORAN 50 WP	chloroxuron	Misc.

Alphabetical list of trade names or active ingredients	Active Ingredient(s)	Relevant Diagnosis and Treatment Section
Terbacil		Misc.
Terbufos		4
Terbuthylazine		16
Terbutryne		16
TERPAL	ethephon + mepiquat chloride	Misc. + 11
TERRA-SYTAM	dimefox	4
Tetrachlorvinphos		4
Tetradifon		Misc.
TETRALEX-PLUS	dicamba + mecoprop + MCPA	12
Tetramethrin		10
Tetrasul		Misc.
TETROXONE M	bromoxynil + ioxynil + dichlorprop + MCPA	2 + 12
Thiabendazole		Misc.
THIMET	phorate	4
Thiofanox		5
Thiometon		4
Thionazin		4
Thiophanate-methyl		Misc.
THIODAN	endosulfan	3
THIOVIT	sulphur	Misc.
Thiram		15
TIEZENE	zineb	15
TILT	propiconazole	Misc.
TIPOFF	NAA (1-naphthylacetic acid)	Misc.
TITAN	chlormequat	Misc.
TOK E-25	nitrofen	Misc.
TOLKAN A	dinoterb + isoproturon	1 + Misc.
TOLKAN LIQUID	isoproturon	Misc.
Tolylfluanid		Misc.
TOPLAWN	2,4-D + fenoprop	12 + Misc.
TOPROSE MILDEW SPRAY	dinocap	1
TOPROSE SYSTEMIC SPRAY	formothion	4
TORAK	dialifos	4
TORDON	picloram	12
TORNADO	acephate	4
TORQUE	fenbutatin oxide	13
TOTRIL	ioxynil	2
TOXAPHENE	camphechlor	3
TREFLAN	trifluralin	Misc.
Tri-allate		Misc.
Triadimefon		Misc.

Alphabetical list of trade names or active ingredients	Active Ingredient(s)	Relevant Diagnosis and Treatment Section
Triazophos		4
TRIBUNIL	methabenzthiazuron	Misc.
Tributyltin oxide		13
Tributyltin phosphate		13
Trichloronitromethane		19(e)
Trichlorphon		4
Tridemorph		Misc.
Trietazine		16
Trifluralin		Misc.
TRIFOCIDE LIQUID DNOC	DNOC	1
TRIFOLEX-TRA	MCPA + MCPB	12
Triforine		Misc.
TRIHERBIDE CIPC	chlorpropham	Misc.
TRIHERBIDE IPC	propham	Misc.
TRIMANGOL 80	maneb	15
TRIOXONE 50	2,4,5-T	12
TRIPOMOL 80	thiram	15
TRITOFTOROL	zineb	15
TROJAN SC	chloridazon	Misc.
TUGON	trichlorphon	4
TURBAIR ROVRAL	iprodione	Misc.
TWIN-TAK	bromoxynil + ioxynil + isoproturon	2 + Misc.
TWINKILL	methazole + simazine	Misc. + 16
UNDENE	propoxur	5
ULVAIR	dioxacarb	5
Vamidothion		4
VAPAM	metham sodium	15
VAPONA	dichlorvos	4
VAPONA FLYKILLER	dichlorvos	4
VARITOX	TCA	Misc.
VECTAL SC	atrazine	16
VEGETABLE PEST & DISEASE DUSTER	rotenone + trichlorphon	4
VELPAR	hexazinone	Misc.
VELVAS	ferrous sulphate	Misc.
VELVETONE LAWN CONDIT. WITH SELECTIVE WK	2,4-D + dicamba	12
VENZAR	lenacil	Misc.
VERDONE	2,4-D + mecoprop	12

Alphabetical list of trade names or active ingredients	Active Ingredient(s)	Relevant Diagnosis and Treatment Section
VERGEMASTER	2,4-D	12
VIGIL	dichlobutrazol	Misc.
VIGIL K	carbendazim + dichlobutrazol	Misc.
VIGON-F	DNOC	1
VIGON-P	MCPA	12
Vinclozolin		Misc.
VITAFUME	metham sodium	15
VITAVAX	carboxin	15
VITAX GREENFLY/ BLACKFLY SPRAY	malathion + dimethoate	4
VITAX LAWN SAND	ferrous sulphate	Misc.
VITAX LAWN WEEDKILLER	2,4-D + mecoprop	12
VOLCK	mineral oil	Misc.
VONDALHYD	maleic hydrazide	Misc.
VONDOZEB	manganese and zinc dithiocarbamate	15
VYDATE	oxamyl	5
Warfarin		18
WASPEND	pirimiphos-methyl + pyrethrins	4 + 10
WEEDAZIN	aminotriazole + simazine	Misc. + 16
WEEDAZOL T-L	aminotriazole	Misc.
WEEDEX	simazine	16
WEEDEX S2G	simazine	16
WEEDOL	paraquat + diquat	11
XLALL INSECTICIDE	nicotine	14
YALTOX	carbofuran	5
Zineb		15
ZINOFOS	thionazin	4
Ziram		15
ZOLONE LIQUID	phosalone	4

Diagnosis and Treatment

1. Dinitro Compounds

Uses
The best known compounds in this group are dinitro-ortho-cresol (DNOC) and dinoseb (DNBP). Dinoseb is used mainly for weed control in young leguminous crops (eg peas and beans), and for potato haulm desiccation. DNOC is used as winter wash for fruit trees and also has a very limited use as a cereal herbicide.

Routes of Absorption
The skin is the common route of absorption, but the prolonged inhalation of spray mist or dust can also cause poisoning.

Pharmacology
These compounds uncouple oxidative phosphorylation. This affects energy transfer at the cellular level and the first reaction is a stimulation of metabolism which is independent of the thyroid gland. The action, if not immediately overwhelming, is rapidly and completely reversible. No tissue damage is produced and the compounds are rapidly broken down and eliminated. DNOC and dinoseb are intense yellow dyes and the other dinitro compounds show this characteristic to a varying degree. The yellow colour in the blood may persist for some time and provide useful evidence of exposure.

Features of Toxicity
The skin and hair may be stained yellow. Anything more than a pale yellow staining of the hands suggests overexposure and indicates that methods of handling should be reviewed to ensure that the recommendations for safe use are being observed.

The main early symptoms of poisoning are fatigue, excessive and unusual sweating and thirst. Insomnia and loss of weight occur in more chronic cases. The symptoms may be erroneously attributed to other causes, eg heat and long hours of work, but when they are present the patient should be promptly removed from possible further exposure to dinitro compounds pending the result of a blood examination. Serious illness may develop rapidly following continued exposure with the patient showing rapidly increasing anxiety and restlessness together with an increased rate and depth of respiration, tachycardia and usually a rise in temperature. Death can occur from exhaustion.

Treatment
Where exposure has occurred all clothing that might be contaminated should be removed at once and exposed areas of skin (hands, arms, face and neck) thoroughly washed with soap and water.

Management of Severe Cases
Any case showing symptoms should be admitted to hospital. No specific treatment for poisoning by dinitro compounds is known and general measures should be used to deal with symptoms as they arise. This includes the continuous administration of oxygen, replacement of fluids and cold sponging or spraying. Absolute rest is essential. Do not give morphine or barbiturates. Once begun, recovery is rapid and complete, but yellow staining of skin and hair persists for days or weeks.

Management of Minor Cases
In a case of symptomless over-exposure, particularly with marked yellow staining of the skin, where, for example, a blood test shows that the concentration of the dinitro compound is between 10 and 20 µg/ml of blood (for determination of dinitro levels see under Laboratory Diagnosis below), the person concerned should be specially supervised to ensure that all the recognised precautions for use are being observed. Another blood specimen should be taken 48 hours later and if the dinitro concentration is higher the worker should be removed immediately from further contact until the blood level has fallen below 5 µg/ml.

If, at an initial examination, the blood dinitro concentration is more than 20 µg/ml the worker must be removed immediately from further exposure to dinitro compounds and not allowed to use them or similar compounds until the level has fallen below 5 µg/ml.

Laboratory Diagnosis
The simple blood test used for the detection of dinitro compounds can be carried out through the London National Poisons Information Service (page i). For this purpose, 5 ml of venous blood should be placed in a tube containing an anti-coagulant (eg heparin) and gently rotated. Postal instructions are given in Appendix III.

The laboratory services can be used for the determination of the dinitro content of blood specimens taken either as a routine precaution or in cases of suspected poisoning.

2. Other Uncouplers Of Oxidative Phosphorylation

Uses
The main chemicals in this group are bromoxynil, ioxynil and pentachlorophenol. Bromoxynil and ioxynil are herbicides which are widely used on cereal crops in the spring and autumn. Ioxynil also has a minor use in horticulture. Pentachlorophenol is used as a fungicide and insecticide in timber treatment, as a fungicide in masonry treatment and as a pre-crop emergence and defoliant herbicide.

Routes of Absorption
The skin is the common route of absorption but the prolonged inhalation of spray mist or dust may increase the risks of poisoning.

Pharmacology
An uncoupling of oxidative phosphorylation with consequent stimulation of cellular metabolism is the major biochemical effect produced by this group of compounds and the action is indistinguishable from that produced by the dinitro compounds. The effect, if not fatal, is rapidly reversible and no lasting physical lesions are produced.

Toxic Effects
Severe and fatal poisoning by pentachlorophenol has been reported in hot countries and a high environmental temperature would be expected to aggravate the hazards from exposure to any of these compounds. Poisoning of humans by ioxynil and bromoxynil has not been reported.

Unlike the dinitro compounds the chemicals in this group are not brightly coloured and therefore staining of the skin cannot be relied upon as evidence of exposure. The main early symptoms of poisoning by pentachlorophenol include fatigue, excessive and unusual sweating and thirst; insomnia and loss of weight may occur in more protracted cases. Serious illness may develop rapidly with further exposure to pentachlorophenol and can prove fatal. The patient shows rapidly increasing anxiety and restlessness, together with an increased rate and depth of respiration, tachycardia and usually a rise of temperature. Although no accidents have been reported with other compounds in this group, similar symptoms may be expected on theoretical grounds.

Treatment
Where exposure has occurred all clothing that might be contaminated should be removed at once and exposed areas of skin (hands, arms, face and neck) thoroughly washed with soap and cold water.

Management of severe cases
Where clinical symptoms are obvious the patient should be sent to hospital. No specific treatment is known at the present time and general measures should be used to deal with symptoms as they arise. Treatment by the continuous administration of oxygen, replacement of fluids and cold sponging or spraying may be necessary. Absolute rest is essential.

Management of minor cases
Where early ill-defined or non-specific symptoms occur, the patient should be promptly removed from possible further exposure pending the result of a urine test (see below). Such symptoms may be erroneously attributed to other causes, eg heat and long hours of work.

Laboratory Diagnosis
No specific tests exist, but urine from any suspected case of poisoning should be obtained and the Poisons Information Service or the manufacturers consulted regarding its possible examination for urinary metabolites.

3. Organochlorine Compounds

Uses
This group comprises a large number of chemicals such as dicophane (DDT), aldrin, dieldrin, gamma-HCH (Gammexane, lindane, gamma-BHC) chlordane, endrin and endosulfan. Over recent years the use of most of these pesticides has been drastically curtailed because they are generally characterised by their persistence in human and animal tissues and in the environment.

Routes of Absorption
The skin is an important route of absorption.

Pharmacology and Toxic Effects
The only known action of organochlorine compounds in acute overdosage is upon the central nervous system. Apprehension and excitement usually occurs a few hours after exposure with fibrillation of the skeletal muscles leading to tremors and convulsions. Initially, respiration is accelerated but later respiratory depression and then apnoea may supervene. These effects may be delayed for up to 48 hours following exposure.

Management and Treatment
When skin contamination has occurred the clothing should be removed as soon as possible and the contaminated area washed thoroughly with soap and cold water. If acute poisoning is associated with ingestion the stomach should be emptied and a saline purgative may be administered though vomiting is contra-indicated if a hydrocarbon solvent is present. Milk or fats (eg olive oil) must NOT be given, because they may enhance the absorption of the pesticide.

Treatment is symptomatic and aimed at controlling convulsions and restoring and maintaining respiration.

To control convulsions the drug of choice is diazepam given intravenously. This treatment may have to be maintained for some days.

Maintenance of pulmonary ventilation may require intubation and mechanical measures.

Once the acute stage is passed, complete recovery, without sequelae, is the rule.

4. Organophosphorus Compounds

Uses
Numerous organophosphorus pesticides of varying toxicity are used extensively in agriculture and horticulture (including glasshouse crops) mainly as emulsifiable concentrates or wettable powder formulations for making up into liquid sprays, but also as granules for soil application. A limited number are also available as fogging formulations, smokes or impregnated resin strip preparations for use indoors.

Routes of Absorption
Absorption may take place via the skin or by inhalation.

Pharmacology
The acute toxicity, speed and duration of effect vary greatly from one organophosphate to another but they all have the same basic mode of toxic action, namely the depression of cholinesterase activity in blood, brain and most other tissues. This effect allows acetylcholine to accumulate at the autonomic and some central synapses, and at the autonomic post-ganglionic and skeletal efferent nerve endings thus blocking the transmission of nerve impulses.

Toxic Effects
The toxic effects are similar to those of a cholinergic drug such as neostigmine, but tend to be much more prolonged, lasting for a day or two rather than a few hours. Successive hours or days of unsafe use may cause progressive depletion of cholinesterase reserves until toxic effects occur. Their onset and severity depend mainly on the speed and degree of cholinesterase depression.

The first symptoms of poisoning are usually a feeling of exhaustion, weakness, and possibly mental confusion. These effects may be experienced during exposure, or up to 12 hours later, and could well be ignored by a person using organophosphorus compounds. Vomiting, cramp-like abdominal pain, excessive cold sweating and salivation may soon follow.

Constriction of one or both pupils and a sensation of tightness in the chest during inspiration may also occur at an early stage but these signs are not reliable indices of the severity of the systemic poisoning because they may be caused by local anti-cholinesterase effects of spray mist in the eye or bronchi.

As poisoning progresses muscular twitchings begin in the eyelids and tongue and then other muscles of the face and neck become involved. Severely affected persons develop generalised muscular twitchings with severe muscular weakness and convulsions may also occur. Miosis is prominent and progressive. Later effects may include diarrhoea, tenesmus, incontinence, ataxia and mental confusion. Bronchial hypersecretion with broncho-constriction and cyanosis lead to respiratory depression and mental confusion, gradually advancing to coma and death from respiratory failure. The clinical picture in very severe cases is one of muscular twitching, profuse sweating, incontinence, mental confusion and progressive cardiac and respiratory failure.

Symptomless depression of cholinesterase levels may render a person much more susceptible to the action of depolarising muscle relaxants, such as succinylcholine, given in conjunction with anaesthesia. In these cases a degree of exposure to organophosphorus compounds which would normally only cause mild clinical poisoning can precipitate a more severe level of poisoning.

Management and Treatment

All cases of organophosphate poisoning should be dealt with as an emergency and the patient admitted to hospital as quickly as possible. A clear airway should be ensured, oxygenation maintained, any necessary skin decontamination carried out and atropine sulphate given as soon as possible in a dose of 2 mg by subcutaneous or intramuscular injection, or in severe cases by the intravenous route. The patient must not be allowed or made to exert himself in any way as muscular exertion may hasten the course of poisoning by inducing more acetylcholine accumulation.

Ventilation must be maintained. In severe cases, especially if treatment has been delayed, there may be excessive mucous secretion, combined with broncho-constriction. Care must therefore be taken to keep the airway clear and it may be necessary to pass an endotracheal tube. There is ample evidence that the immediate treatment of respiratory arrest by aspiration of bronchial secretions and assisted ventilation may permit full recovery.

As the skin is the commonest route of absorption thorough decontamination is essential. All clothing that is, or might be, contaminated should be removed at once, and all possibly contaminated skin washed thoroughly with soap and cold water including exposed areas (eg hands, arms, face, neck and hair).

Two specific antidotes exist for use in organophosphorus compound poisoning. Atropine antagonises the so-called muscarinic effects of accumulating acetylcholine and may therefore considerably improve the patient's condition. Certain oxime compounds, notably pralidoxime, are able rapidly to reverse the inhibition of cholinesterase enzymes by some (but not all — see product label) organophosphorus compounds and may thus reverse the course of poisoning provided that they are given promptly after exposure has occurred.

In mild cases one injection of atropine may be enough to relieve symptoms, but if not, further atropine sulphate in 2 mg doses should be given at frequent intervals (15-30 minutes), until the patient is fully atropinised, ie dilated pupils, dry mouth and rapid pulse. Persons suffering from organophosphate poisoning tolerate more atropine than do normal persons. Very large amounts, 100 mg or more, may be required to maintain atropinisation and control symptoms throughout the course of poisoning. The heart rate is a particularly useful criterion in the use of atropine and a target rate for the first 24 hours is 80 beats per minute. At 24 hours the need for atropine should be reviewed.

In addition, diazepam by separate intravenous injection in doses of 5-10 mg, appears to have a beneficial, non-specific effect, apart from controlling tremors or convulsions. If a cholinesterase reactivator, eg pralidoxime, is available within 12 hours of the onset of symptoms it should be given intramuscularly or intravenously as early as possible, in any severe or progressive case of intoxication. Treatment by both atropine and pralidoxime should be carried out at the same time as the two methods are complementary. (If the reactivator is effective, the symptoms will be promptly controlled, and further atropine will probably not be needed). For slowly metabolised indirect inhibitors of cholinesterase it may sometimes be necessary to repeat both pralidoxime and atropine even after 24 hours.

In Britain, the oxime reactivator available is pralidoxime which can be obtained on demand from certain strategic depots (see Appendix IV). The dose is 1g pralidoxime, dissolved in 2-3 ml of water for intramuscular, or 6-20 ml water for intravenous injection. A single dose may be sufficient to control the toxic effects, but in some cases a second or even third dose per 24 hours may be necessary to maintain control. Use of the anticonvulsant diazepam (10 mg by separate intravenous injection repeated as necessary) will often improve the clinical condition.

In summary the management of organophosphate poisoning should be as follows:

1. Maintain oxygenation;

2. Decontaminate the skin thoroughly but gently;

3. Administer atropine sulphate subcutaneously or intravenously and also take a venous blood sample, at the time, into a lithium heparin tube for cholinesterase estimation (see below) if not already taken;

4. Give a cholinesterase reactivator intramuscularly or intravenously and,

5. Repeat 3 and 4 as necessary.

6. Take further blood samples as necessary to monitor recovery.

Laboratory diagnosis
Diagnosis of poisoning by organophosphorus compounds can be confirmed by demonstrating a significantly reduced cholinesterase activity in whole blood, red blood cells, or plasma. A blood test should be made in every suspected case, but only after any emergency resuscitation has been instituted. Ten ml of venous blood should be taken into a lithium heparin tube, avoiding haemolysis and sent to the nearest laboratory equipped for cholinesterase determination (Appendix III).

A significantly reduced level of cholinesterase activity in the red cells indicates that an anti-cholinesterase chemical has been absorbed. A reduction in pseudocholinesterase (plasma) activity merely indicates exposure to such a chemical. If the depression is marked, the patient will be more susceptible to the effects of further exposure to an organophosphorus compound. Any person who has been detectably affected should not, therefore, be allowed to return to work or come into contact with any organophosphorus compound until the level of blood cholinesterase activity has been restored. The rate of recovery of cholinesterase activity in the blood varies with the chemical responsible. Complete recovery in certain circumstances may take two or three months. It is therefore advisable for an affected person to have further blood examinations every 7-14 days until recovery is complete.

Difficulty often arises regarding the interpretation of results of blood tests as individuals vary quite widely in their normal complement of cholinesterase and it may be necessary to seek expert advice. Ideally, those likely to be repeatedly engaged with handling organophosphorus compounds, eg pilots involved in aerial spraying, contract sprayers on the ground, should have a baseline estimation carried out before starting on this work.

5. Carbamates

This section refers only to insecticidal (anticholinesterase) carbamates and not to other types of carbamates, such as those used as herbicides.

Uses
There are a number of compounds in this group used in agriculture and horticulture as insecticidal and nematicidal preparations whilst insecticidal preparations are used in food storage, animal husbandry and public hygiene practice. Carbamates are also incorporated in preparations for use in both home and garden.

Routes of Absorption
Carbamates are generally and readily absorbed by inhalation and through the skin, as well as by ingestion. They can also have local effects on the eyes.

Pharmacology and Toxic Effects
The acute toxicity, speed and duration of effect, of which there is great variation between the separate carbamates, is influenced by the chemical structure. All of these compounds nevertheless have the same basic mode of toxic action, namely the depression of cholinesterase activity in blood, brain and most other tissues. The resulting accumulation of acetylcholine at synapses and nerve endings blocks the transmission of nerve impulses.

The toxic effects are therefore similar to those of the organophosphorus insecticides, but both onset and recovery are markedly more rapid. Prolonged or repeated unsafe use can result in progressive depletion of cholinesterase reserves until toxic effects occur. Their onset and severity depend mainly on both the speed and degree of cholinesterase depression.

The symptomatology of poisoning by anticholinesterase agents is described in detail in the section on organophosphorus compounds. Early signs are headache and nausea followed by a sensation of tightness in the chest, coughing and constriction of the pupils. As poisoning progresses muscular twitching occurs and becomes generalised, and there may be marked central nervous or gastro-intestinal manifestations. Poisoning by carbamates may also cause circulatory failure, dyspnoea, hypopnoea and marked bradycardia. The clinical picture in a severe case is one of muscular twitching, profuse sweating, incontinence, mental confusion and progressive cardiac and respiratory failure.

Symptomless depression of cholinesterase levels increases susceptibility to the action of depolarising muscle relaxants such as succinylcholine given in conjunction with anaesthesia and can give rise to severe poisoning with other anticholinesterase agents at levels of exposure which would normally only produce mild clinical effects.

Management and Treatment
All cases of carbamate poisoning should be dealt with as an emergency. The patient must not be allowed or made to exert himself in any way as muscular exertion may hasten the course of poisoning by inducing more acetylcholine accumulation. A clear airway should be ensured, adequate oxygenation maintained, any necessary decontamination carried out and atropine sulphate given as soon as possible in a dose of 2 mg by subcutaneous or intramuscular injection, or in severe cases by the intravenous route, to reverse the signs of poisoning. The patient should be admitted to hospital as quickly as possible.

Respiratory failure is the usual cause of death. If respiratory depression occurs, ventilation must be maintained. There may be excessive mucous secretion combined with broncho-constriction and care must be taken to maintain a clear airway; it may sometimes be necessary to pass an endotracheal tube. Prompt treatment of respiratory arrest by aspiration of bronchial secretions and assisted ventilation is essential.

All clothing that is, or might be, contaminated should be removed at once and all possibly contaminated skin washed thoroughly with soap and cold water especially the exposed areas of hands, arms, face, neck and hair. If there have been splashes in the eyes these should be irrigated with water or physiological saline.

Atropine is the specific antidote for carbamate-induced inhibition of cholinesterase. In mild cases one dose may be sufficient, but if the patient does not respond or continues to develop toxic manifestations further 2 mg doses should be given at frequent intervals (15-30 minutes), using the intravenous route in severe cases until the patient is fully atropinised ie dilated pupils, dry mouth and rapid pulse. Pralidoxime has little, if any, value in the treatment of carbamate over-exposure and should not be used for this purpose.

Laboratory Diagnosis
Diagnosis of poisoning by carbamates can be confirmed by demonstrating a significantly reduced cholinesterase activity in whole blood, red blood cells or plasma. A blood test should be made in every suspected case. 10 ml of venous blood should be placed in a lithium heparin tube, avoiding haemolysis, and sent to the nearest laboratory equipped for cholinesterase determination (Appendix III), as quickly as possible (within 1-4 hours). Because of the rapid reactivation of cholinesterases inhibited by carbamate compounds it is not recommended to send such samples by post.

6. Fluoroacetic Acid Derivatives

Uses
In Britain the use of fluoroacetic acid derivatives is now confined to that of a rodenticide in ships' holds and sewers.

Routes of Absorption
There is little toxic danger from these compounds unless they are taken into the mouth.

Pharmacology
Fluoroacetic acid compounds inhibit energy transformation by blocking the tricarboxylic acid cycle. The brain and the heart are primarily affected. The acute lethal dose may be as little as 30 mg for an adult.

Toxic Effects
The onset of symptoms following absorption by the percutaneous or oral routes is characteristically delayed for 30 minutes to 2 hours, or even longer. Nausea and apprehension develop, followed by muscle twitching, tremors, cardiac irregularities, convulsions and coma. Death occurs from respiratory and cardiac failure, often associated with pulmonary oedema.

Management and Treatment
Contaminated clothing should be removed and the affected skin washed thoroughly with soap and cold water. If the chemical has been swallowed the stomach should be emptied as soon as possible.

Ensure a clear airway and maintain respiration. No specific antidote is known for man. Hypocalcaemia may occur and serum calcium levels should be monitored. Convulsions and cardiac dysrhythmias may respond to intravenous calcium gluconate. If necessary convulsions should be controlled with intravenous diazepam.

Laboratory Diagnosis
Few laboratories are able to conduct specific tests for fluoroacetates but specimens of blood, faeces and urine should be retained in a deep freeze for possible forensic purposes.

7. Organic Mercurials

Uses
Phenyl mercury acetate — an aryl (cyclic) compound — is used in both dry and liquid seed treatments and methoxyethyl mercury acetate — an alkyl (non-cyclic) compound is used in liquid seed treatments. In addition aryl mercury compounds can be used as foliage sprays and in canker paints, whilst ethyl mercury phosphate, (an alkyl compound) phenyl mercury catechol (an aryl compound) and methoxyethylmercury chloride (an alkyl compound) are used as dips or steeps for seeds or bulbs.

Routes of Absorption
Organic mercurial pesticides can be absorbed by inhalation or through the skin.

Pharmacology and Toxic Effects
Organic mercurials combine with sulphydryl (SH) groups and it is assumed that the toxic effects in man are due to interference with enzymes having such chemical groupings but the precise mode of action is unknown.

The aryl compounds are much less toxic to man than the alkyl and alkoxy compounds. The latter penetrate rapidly to the central nervous system, where they act selectively on the area striata, the granule-cell layer of the neo-cerebellum and the posterior spinal roots and posterior column.

Acute topical exposure to organic mercury compounds may cause burns of the skin, with redness and blistering after 6-12 hours. Although a single dermal exposure is unlikely to lead to systemic poisoning, mercury has been found in the blister fluid, and it is recommended that blisters should be drained.

Exposure to organo-mercurials in the air causes irritation of the mucous membranes of the eyes and upper respiratory tract and acute systemic poisoning resulting in gastro-intestinal symptoms and renal damage.

These compounds may be absorbed through the skin but once in the body alkyl compounds are distributed differently in the tissues from aryl mercury compounds and cause damage to the central nervous system. Chronic exposure leads to fatigue, impairment of memory, inability to concentrate, numbness and tingling of the lips, fingers and toes; such symptoms often develop insidiously. The physical signs of neurological disturbances are remarkably varied. Tremor and slight ataxia may be the only early signs. In advanced cases, however, severe generalised ataxia, dysarthria and tunnel vision may be totally disabling.

There is no evidence that the aryl compounds affect the central nervous system.

Management and Treatment
Skin splashes should be treated immediately by washing thoroughly. Contaminated clothing must be removed and all contaminated areas of the skin washed with soap and water.

In acute poisoning by ingestion the stomach should be emptied.

Wherever it is available, N-acetyl penicillamine is the drug of choice and has proved to be particularly effective in many cases of chronic mercury poisoning. Alternatively, penicillamine or dimercaprol (BAL) may be given. Examples of suitable regimes are as follows:

N-acetyl penicillamine:	250 mg four times daily by mouth for a period of up to 10 days.
penicillamine:	as for N-acetyl penicillamine
dimercaprol (BAL):	300 mg by deep intramuscular injection at once followed by 200 mg every four hours for 24 hours. Therapy on the following days will be dependant on the severity of poisoning and should be up to 200 mg twice daily for up to 7 days. Injections of dimercaprol are painful and locally irritant and should be given by deep intramuscular injection at different sites.

Laboratory Diagnosis
The estimation of mercury in urine collected over twenty-four hours may be of value in confirming that mercury has been absorbed. However, because of delayed excretion significantly raised levels may not be found until a week or more following exposure. Facilities for mercury estimations are provided by the National Poisons Information Service (see page i for address/telephone number and Appendix III for postal instructions).

8. Inorganic Mercurials

Uses
Mercurous chloride can be used as a fungicide. It is applied as a dust, dip or drench on onion seed, shallots and transplants or to brassica transplants. It is also a constituent of some lawn sands. Mercuric oxide can be used as a canker paint on apples and pears (including home garden use).

Routes of Absorption
Poisoning by inorganic mercury compounds is more likely to arise from accidental or intentional ingestion rather than through absorption from the skin.

Toxic Effects

Mercuric oxide is highly toxic and causes coagulation, irritation and superficial corrosion of the tissues with which it comes into contact. Thus, if ingested, it has a rapid action on the mucosa throughout the gastro-intestinal tract. Acute poisoning by mercuric oxide follows accidental or intentional ingestion. Quantities of 0.5g give rise to symptoms of poisoning and higher doses can be fatal.

Earlier symptoms include an astringent or metallic taste and salivation with swelling and ashy discoloration of the mucous membranes of the mouth and pharynx. Intense thirst and abdominal pain with vomiting of blood-stained shreds of mucus follow whilst diarrhoea, often bloody, may be profuse. Circulatory collapse may occur at an early stage.

If the acute reaction is survived albuminuria and anuria may still occur, with a fatal outcome.

Mercurous chloride is much less toxic but a few cases have been reported of circulatory collapse and death in persons who have taken calomel in large quantities.

Management and Treatment
Although percutaneous absorption is usually insignificant it is prudent to remove clothing that might be contaminated and wash the skin and hair thoroughly. Unless vigorous spontaneous vomiting has taken place the stomach should be emptied by emesis or gastric aspiration. Management should be directed to energetic measures to counteract shock.

For therapy, see under ORGANIC MERCURIALS p. 50

Laboratory Diagnosis
The presence of more than 100 µg of mercury in the urine collected over 24 hours indicates absorption but not necessarily poisoning. Persistent albuminuria in a person using inorganic mercury compounds should be considered to be caused by the absorption of mercury until other possible causes have been excluded. For laboratory facilities see under Organic Mercurials p. 50.

9. Arsenical Compounds

Uses
Arsenical pesticide formulations are now restricted to the very small scale use of copper acetoarsenite in agriculture and horticulture, arsenious oxide used as an acute rodenticide and copper, chrome and arsenic formulations for the pre-treatment of timber. As these substances are highly toxic, prompt diagnosis and treatment are essential.

Routes of Absorption
Absorption takes place rapidly from the gastro-intestinal tract and can also occur, although at a lower rate, via the respiratory tract and through the skin.

Pharmacology
Most arsenicals are irritants and also cause dilation and increased permeability of blood capillaries. At the cellular level arsenic combines with sulphydryl groups thereby inhibiting the action of certain enzymes eg keto acid oxidases.

Toxic Effects
The intake of arsenicals by any route, but notably after ingestion, induces a characteristically sudden onset of abdominal pain and vomiting. This usually occurs about half an hour after ingestion although the interval may be longer. Diarrhoea, often profuse, may follow and a 'choleraic' state may then arise, with profound dehydration, severe hypotension and gross electrolyte disturbance. Hyponatraemia and hypokalaemia may ensue and give rise to muscle cramps in the abdomen and limbs. Death may come about if the electrolyte disturbance is not promptly and fully corrected or may occur as the result of the cellular enzyme disturbance. Death is often presaged by ECG changes.

Repeated exposure to sub-lethal amounts may lead to chronic

poisoning characterised by anorexia, weight loss, diarrhoea, peripheral neuritis and skin rash of the distinctive and so-called 'rain-drop' type.

Treatment
Contaminated clothing should be removed and the skin washed thoroughly. If the arsenic has been swallowed, gastric lavage is indicated only when vomiting has not occurred.

Therapy is the same as for Organic Mercurials (see pg 50).

Prompt administration of the antidote is essential in cases of acute arsenical poisoning.

Laboratory Diagnosis
Circumstantial evidence usually gives the clue to arsenical poisoning. This can be confirmed by chemical analysis of the vomitus or faeces for arsenic. Samples should always be kept carefully for this purpose.

In chronic poisoning a raised level of arsenic may be found in the hair and nails but only a few laboratories are equipped for making reliable estimations.

10. Pyrethrins and Synthetic Pyrethroids

This group of pesticides is increasingly widely used in agricultural, horticultural, food storage, animal husbandry and public hygiene practice as well as in the home. They are used mainly as contact or 'knockdown' insecticides (ie with immediate action) although some recently developed pyrethroids also possess residual activity. Both pyrethrins and synthetic pyrethroids are often used in conjunction with other chemicals which enhance their effectiveness.

Routes of Absorption
The skin and especially the lungs are regarded as being the likely routes of absorption.

Pharmacology and Toxic Effects
Whilst natural pyrethrins have a low oral toxicity to mammals, the synthetic pyrethroids exhibit a wide degree of oral toxicity ranging from the relatively non-toxic bioresmethrin to the highly toxic decamethrin. The dermal toxicities of both pyrethrins and synthetic pyrethroids are, however, very low such that systemic toxicity from such exposure does not represent a hazard.

The probable mode of action of this group of pesticides is on the central nervous system by blocking the transmission of nerve impulses. Acute toxic effects have not been seen in man but in animals they include excitation, tetanic convulsions and muscular fibrillation with death from respiratory or circulatory failure.

Management and Treatment
The low toxicity of pyrethrins and of some synthetic pyrethroids means that the intake of dangerous doses in these cases is low. However, for the more toxic synthetic pyrethroids or where large quantities of pyrethrins or pyrethroids of low toxicity are thought to

have been ingested and there is evidence of poisoning, the gastrointestinal tract should be cleared by gastric lavage and purgation, a forced diuresis established and symptomatic and supportive measures applied as necessary. If there are convulsions or muscular fibrillation, diazepam should be used.

11. Bipyridilium Compounds

Uses
The non-selective herbicides paraquat and diquat are the principal members of this group used commercially. Paraquat is the more effective against grasses and is widely used for general weed control, in the renovation of pasture, as an alternative to ploughing before sowing a new crop, and in the garden as a "chemical hoe". Diquat is more effective against broad-leaved weeds and is used for the dessication of potato haulm before harvesting and often in combination with paraquat for the suppression of weeds after sowing and before the emergence of a crop. Liquid concentrates of paraquat and diquat (10-20 per cent ions w/w) are available for agricultural and industrial uses but are not intended for use by the home gardener. For such uses paraquat and diquat are combined in a solid formulation (5 per cent total bipyridilium ions w/w).

Routes of Absorption
Only very small quantities are absorbed through the skin or by inhalation. The major risk of poisoning arises from either inadvertent or deliberate ingestion.

Pharmacology
Paraquat is used either as the dichloride or dimethosulphate salt; diquat is used as the dibromide salt. The pharmacological and toxic effects are due to the cations — the salts being fully dissociated in solution. From an oral dose the amount absorbed is variable and not accurately known for man. Attempts to estimate the amounts ingested from the amounts excreted in urine are of doubtful value. Of the total amount excreted in the urine more than 90 per cent is eliminated within 48 hours although total excretion is usually prolonged. From large single doses paraquat may behave as a direct toxic agent in a number of tissues notably the lung, liver or kidneys.

Toxic Effects

Ingestion

The immediate effects of ingestion are similar with both compounds and are due to their local irritant action on mucous membranes. Vomiting, abdominal discomfort and diarrhoea are followed by soreness of the mouth and throat, and difficulty in swallowing. Massive doses may produce rapid multi-organ failure and death within 24-48 hours. Following the ingestion of smaller quantities, signs of kidney and liver damage may appear within the first one to three days, although this damage is spontaneously reversible. Signs of pulmonary dysfunction may also develop after a few days even in the absence of immediate signs of local irritant action. Pulmonary function tests may be abnormal before clinical signs of lung damage are obvious. The onset of dypsnoea is an indication of a poor prognosis. Subsequently there may be pulmonary oedema and, with paraquat only, the development of progressive pulmonary fibrosis with death due to respiratory insufficiency.

Several cases of systemic poisoning with diquat have been reported in man. Changes similar to those seen with paraquat were recorded except that there was no evidence of pulmonary fibrosis.

Skin contact

Paraquat and diquat have local irritant effects particularly on eye or mucous membranes. Splashes left in contact with the skin for any length of time cause irritation and inflammation. In severe cases blister formation may occur. There is considerable individual variation in the skin response to the bipyridyls. Concentrated solution of either compound remaining in contact with the base of the nail lead to transverse cracking followed by shedding of the nail. With minor contamination, white spots may occur in the nail which eventually grow out. Histologically the spots consist of areas where the epithelial structure has been preserved instead of being transformed into keratin in the formation of nail. When the nail is shed the subsequent regrowth of normal nail follows without delay.

Contact of solutions with cuts or wounds of the skin leads to delay in healing. Contact of solid with mucous membranes of the lips causes soreness and, in some cases, blister formation. Deaths from systemic paraquat poisoning have been described after skin exposure from leaking spray containers, etc, but these remain to be validated.

Eyes

Splashes of liquid concentrate in the eyes may lead to severe inflammation which develops gradually and reaches its maximum at 12-24 hours. There may be extensive stripping of superficial areas of corneal and conjunctival epithelium. Although healing may be slow the injury is usually superficial and, even in severe cases, recovery is often complete, given proper medical care. All cases of conjunctival irritation after 24 hours should be seen by an eye specialist.

Inhalation

Inhalation of spray mist or dust of paraquat or diquat causes epistaxis. Normally, however, only a very small proportion of spray consists of drops of a diameter within the respirable range and the risk of bronchopulmonary damage in this manner is remote. Thus, in the course of spraying operations using correct techniques there is negligible risk of poisoning from inhalation.

Management and Treatment

Ingestion

Deaths have occurred in people ingesting quite small amounts of paraquat concentrate (probably 10-15 ml). The onset of serious symptoms may be delayed for 2-3 days after the incident. Every case should be referred immediately to hospital, where the particular formulation ingested should be ascertained and the presence of paraquat or diquat in urine confirmed by analysis (see Laboratory Diagnosis). Several medical centres throughout England and Wales have agreed on a comprehensive scheme to provide treatment in cases of systemic paraquat poisoning. The National Poisons Information Services (telephone numbers listed on page i) can provide the addresses of these medical centres and also of laboratories with appropriate assay facilities. Laboratory facilities exist for radio-immune or colorimetric assay of paraquat in plasma and the results can furnish a valuable prognostic index.

Where paraquat or diquat has been ingested, vomiting should be induced at once, if it has not already occurred, and this should be followed without delay by gastric lavage. However, if treatment is only begun some hours after ingestion, stomach wash-out should be attempted only in hospital as oesophageal ulceration may have occurred. The use of oxygen in the early stages of treatment is contraindicated.

There is no specific antidote to the bipyridyls. Treatment is directed to preventing absorption from the alimentary tract and accelerating the elimination from the body of any bipyridyl ion which has been absorbed. Once gastric lavage has been carried out, and provided there is no evidence of corrosive injury to the throat, absorption may be lessened by introducing into the stomach 100-200ml of a 15-30% suspension of Fullers Earth or bentonite together with 20ml magnesium sulphate solution (Magnesium Sulphate Mixture, BP). (NB. 200ml of a 20% mannitol solution may be used as an alternative to the magnesium sulphate solution). This acts as a purge and adsorbs dipyridylium ions remaining in the gut. Even more effective in minimising absorption is gut irrigation via a nasogastric tube using a 3% suspension of bentonite in normal saline at a rate of 2 litres per hour. This gut irrigation should be continued until the bowel effluent shows no significant concentration of dipyridylium ions (see Laboratory Diagnosis).

Gut irrigation at the rate recommended will also tend to produce an adequate diuresis to promote the renal excretion of the compound which has been absorbed by the body and this avoids the need to institute a separate intravenous fluid load which would otherwise be advisable. Serum electrolytes should be closely monitored during this period. As well as these measures it has been recommended that haemodialysis or haemoperfusion should also be instituted.

The late effects of lung or renal damage which may be caused by these compounds can only be treated symptomatically.

Poisoning from paraquat by ingestion is often associated with suicide and the quantities swallowed deliberately are usually so large that existing methods of treatment are not effective.

Skin contact
Absorption of the bipyridyls through intact skin is minimal at spray dilution. Measurable amounts may however, be absorbed when splashes of the concentrates, or clothing contaminated with the concentrates, remain in contact with the skin, for prolonged periods. To avoid the risk of local inflammation and possible absorption contaminated clothing must be removed as soon as possible and splashes washed off.

Apart from avoidance of further contact, no specific treatment is indicated for epistaxis or injury to the finger nails.

Eye contact
Eye splashes require immediate irrigation followed by treatment with antibiotics to control infection. After regrowth of the corneal and conjunctival epithelium is complete, treatment with a steroid may be necessary to aid the resolution of granulation tissue. Visual acuity may be temporarily impaired for up to three or four weeks by the persistence of corneal oedema. All but the most minor eye injuries should be seen by a specialist at an early stage.

Laboratory Diagnosis
Both paraquat and diquat can readily be determined in urine. Urine analysis will promptly confirm qualitatively that a bipyridyl has been absorbed. The National Poisons Information Service should be consulted at once about plasma level measurements.

12. Phenoxyacetates and Related Compounds

Uses
Phenoxyacetates (MCPA, 2,4-D, 2,4,5-T) and related compounds (mecoprop, dichlorprop, MCPB etc) are very widely used for the selective control of weeds in agriculture and home gardens and by local authorities. Mixtures of these herbicides with themselves and other herbicides are very common.

Routes of Absorption
This may take place through the skin and by inhalation.

Pharmacology
These herbicides act as growth regulating hormones in plants, but their toxic action in animals is poorly understood.

Toxic Effects
Following ingestion, there is burning of the oral mucosa, hypersalivation, stomach cramps, vomiting and diarrhoea. Other reported symptoms include convulsions, cerebral depression and mental confusion, with difficulty in speaking. A short period of myotonia is followed by muscular weakness, a general reduction in motor activity, ataxia and inco-ordination and a gradual loss of reflexes. In severe cases coma may develop, followed by death.

The pulse may be rapid and sometimes irregular with a low blood pressure. Ventricular fibrillation has been reported.

Kidney and liver damage have been reported in animal experiments, but not, so far, in man.

The only known cases of phenoxyacetate poisoning are those from deliberate ingestion and no poisoning arising occupationally has ever been verified.

Management and Treatment
There is no known specific antidote for phenoxyacetates and related compounds.

All clothing that might be contaminated should be removed at once and exposed areas of skin washed with soap and cold water.

If ingestion has occurred vomiting usually follows but, nevertheless, the stomach should be emptied.

ECG monitoring is helpful in severe cases of poisoning.

There is some evidence that the establishment of forced alkaline diuresis may substantially augment excretion of 2, 4-D and, to a lesser extent, mecoprop and so contribute to a more favourable prognosis.

13. Organotin Compounds

Uses
Triphenyltin (fentin) compounds, viz the acetate and hydroxide, are used as contact fungicides on potatoes.

Routes of Absorption
Although triphenyltin is very toxic when given parenterally, it appears to be poorly absorbed from the gastro-intestinal tract and also does not pass readily through unbroken skin.

Pharmacology and Toxic Effects
Once absorbed triphenyltin is only very slowly excreted. Although much is known about its effects on biochemical systems in vitro the mechanisms of its toxicity has not yet been explained. The effects of triphenyltin are quite different from those of diphenyltin which acts mainly as an irritant. Symptoms include depression, lethargy, unsteadiness, weakness, moderate diarrhoea and anorexia.

Management and Treatment
No specific antidote is known.

Contaminated clothing should be removed and exposed areas of the skin washed with soap and cold water. If triphenyltin is accidentally swallowed vomiting should be induced and the stomach washed out with 5% sodium bicarbonate if available. Apart from this, treatment is symptomatic.

Laboratory Diagnosis
There is no specific test for triphenyltin poisoning.

14. Nicotine

Uses
Nicotine is now used on a small scale almost exclusively in glasshouses, usually as a smoke (ie nicotine shreds) and occasionally as a spray.

Routes of Absorption
Absorption can occur rapidly through the skin, by inhalation or by ingestion.

Pharmacology
The effects of nicotine result chiefly from its action on the autonomic ganglia and as little as 40 mg pure nicotine can prove lethal.

Toxic Effects
Initially nausea, dizziness, vomiting, respiratory stimulation, headache, tachycardia, sweating and salivation occur followed by prostration, convulsions, cardiac irregularities and coma. Death may supervene within minutes or be delayed for a few hours.

Management and Treatment
Contaminated clothing should be removed and the skin thoroughly washed with soap and cold water. If nicotine has been swallowed, the stomach should be emptied and a purgative administered.

There is no specific antidote. Convulsions should be controlled with diazepam, an airway ensured and respiration maintained.

If death has not occurred within four hours recovery is usually complete.

Laboratory Diagnosis
The levels of nicotine in the plasma may be estimated by gas-liquid chromatography and the National Poisons Information Service should be consulted for advice on this.

15. Dithiocarbamate Fungicides

Uses
Many compounds in this group are used, either alone or in mixtures, as fungicides. They are applied repeatedly to crops as dusts or wettable powders. The most widely used dithiocarbamates are maneb, zineb, and nabam. They are employed mainly in orchards, in glasshouses, on arable crops such as potatoes, and celery, in council allotments and private gardens and as seed-dressings.

Routes of Absorption
Absorption from the gastro-intestinal tract is limited.

Pharmacology
The acute oral toxicity of dithiocarbamate fungicides is low. Some liberation of carbon disulphide is believed to occur during metalobic degradation in the gut, or after absorption. There are no reports of fatal poisoning in man.

Toxic Effects
Despite their very wide use in industry and agriculture the only ill-effects reported from the normal use of the dithiocarbamates have been occasional cases of primary skin or mucosal irritation of a temporary nature. Nausea and vomiting have followed persistent gross over-exposure during manufacture, formulation and packaging. Central nervous system effects without distinctive features are said to occur and these could lead to death from respiratory paralysis. Irritation of the skin and mucosae occur in factory workers but true sensitisation is rare.

Management and Treatment
Acute poisoning with normal use is very unlikely. Gross over-exposure by ingestion is the most likely cause of poisoning in man.

Absorption should be minimised by emptying the stomach and purgation. The amount of absorbed material may be sufficient to cause non-specific central nervous system effects and, possibly, serious respiratory depression. Ventilation must therefore be carefully maintained. There is no known specific antidote and treatment is supportive and symptomatic.

There is no special treatment for skin irritation and sensitisation. Conventional measures are all that are necessary with subsequent protection against exposure.

16. Triazine Herbicides

Uses
The "triazine" chemical series includes a large number of herbicides, eg simazine, atrazine, prometryne, desmetryne, terbutryne, trietazine, cyanazine, terbuthylazine, aziprotryne and others. Their physical and biological properties and their uses vary. At low dosages, the triazines are mainly used for selective weed control in crops, eg beans, peas, cereals, brassicae, fruit trees and many others. At higher doses, certain triazines (particularly simazine and atrazine) are used for the complete control of vegetation on, eg railway tracks, gravel paths, road-edges and playgrounds. Triazine herbicides are usually supplied for dilution with water before use.

Routes of Absorption
Uptake percutaneously and via the lungs is not seen to any great extent.

Pharmacology
The herbicidal triazines are not very soluble in water and are virtually non-volatile. At normal use concentrations they have no recognisable pharmacological effects in animals. Their mode of action in plants is to interfere with photosynthesis so the lack of mammalian response at low concentrations is not surprising. With larger doses toxic effects in animals are slow in onset and non-specific, including weakness, apathy, weight loss, diarrhoea, occasionally laboured respiration, convulsive movements, stupor, then death in coma. Prolonged daily dosage with large but sub-lethal amounts in animals leads to a variety of non-specific pathological effects in the liver, blood-forming tissues, lungs and gastrointestinal tract but there is no well-defined pattern of response.

Toxic Effects
There are no reports of any serious or fatal human poisoning by triazine herbicides, presumably due to their low oral and dermal

toxicity, low water-solubility and a mode of action specific to plant metabolic systems. It is probable that very large doses would have to be ingested to produce toxic effects in man and the effects would be delayed and non-specific. The triazines are not irritant to skin or mucous membranes and no proven case of allergic sensitisation has been reported.

Management and Treatment
Toxic effects are likely to occur only from the ingestion of comparatively large amounts in which case the stomach should be emptied. As there is no known specific antidote, treatment must be symptomatic and supportive.

17. Chlorates

Uses
Sodium chlorate is an oxidising agent which greatly increases the flammability of organic matter (eg clothing) on which it may become deposited. It is used as a weedkiller, mostly for non-selective use, such as in industrial areas and on pathways and drives. The principal risk associated with the handling of chlorates is that of fire or explosion; some serious and, indeed, fatal incidents have occurred.

Routes of Absorption
Absorption does not take place significantly through the skin or via the respiratory tract but can take place following accidental or deliberate ingestion.

Pharmacology
Sodium and potassium chlorates are readily water-soluble and are strong oxidising agents. The chlorate ion is very irritant and, after absorption, converts haemoglobin to methaemoglobin.

Toxic Effects
A dose of about 15g may be fatal for an adult and one of about 2g for a child. Ingestion is followed by vomiting, abdominal pain, confusion, cyanosis, methaemoglobinaemia, haemolysis, convulsions, kidney damage and anuria.

Treatment
Prompt emptying of the stomach is essential, followed by a saline purge and activated charcoal by mouth. Methaemoglobinaemia should be treated by intravenous methylene blue (5 to 24 ml of 1 per cent solution). Fluid intake and output should be maintained as far as possible at 2 to 3 litres in 24 hours. This will aid elimination of

chlorate. Haemolysis may warrant exchange transfusion. For renal damage with oliguria or anuria, haemo dialysis or peritoneal dialysis may be necessary. Although death may be delayed when kidney failure occurs it is usual for recovery to ensue if the patient survives the first 24 hours.

Laboratory Diagnosis
Chlorate may be detected analytically in vomitus, stomach washings or urine.

18. Anticoagulant Rodenticides

Uses
At the present time anticoagulants are the most widely used agents for controlling rats and mice and are also used, in some counties, for controlling grey squirrels in woodlands. Chemically the various examples fall into two main groups — the hydroxycoumarins and the indandione derivatives. Commonly a low concentration of the active ingredient is incorporated in a cereal bait but more concentrated preparations ("master mixes") may be supplied to be diluted before use. They are also used in tracking dusts, in wax-impregnated blocks or as solutions of a soluble salt in water.

All baits contain a distinctively coloured dyestuff as a warning.

Routes of Absorption
There is little risk of anticoagulant rodenticides being absorbed by users and danger arises only when such chemicals are swallowed.

Pharmacology
All of these compounds interfere with the synthesis of prothrombin and related clotting factors by the liver, resulting in a bleeding tendency. The onset of action is commonly delayed and the major effect is achieved by successive doses over a number of days rather than by a single massive dose. However, certain of these compounds are said to produce an acute response but this has not been seen in man. The death of rodents is caused by extensive haemorrhage, usually internally.

Toxic Effects
For a man to be poisoned by the ready-to-use baits, enormous quantities would have to be ingested and, even for the more concentrated preparations, quite large quantities would need to be swallowed. Serious cases in man are virtually unknown except

where deliberate and prolonged administration has been carried out homicidally.

Overdose is exhibited by blood in the urine and faeces, by bruising and by a manifest delay in haemostasis. This is confirmed by a prolongation of the prothrombin time.

Management and Treatment
Vitamin K_1 (phytomenadione) 10-20 mg intramuscular injection, is the specific remedy but daily doses may be necessary until the clotting status returns to normal. In extreme cases the transfusion of fresh frozen plasma or blood may be indicated.

Laboratory Diagnosis
This is based on measurement of the prothrombin time by the usual haematological methods.

19. Fumigants

Although more commonly used for the fumigation of cereals, foodstuffs and other commodities, ships' holds, freight containers, flour mills and food premises infested with insects, mites·or rodents, fumigants are also used for fumigating compost in mushroom houses, soil in greenhouses and for killing rabbits and other vermin outdoors.

19(a). Methyl Bromide

Uses
Methyl bromide is a volatile liquid supplied in gas cylinders and small canisters and is employed as a fumigant in buildings, including warehouses, grain stores and ships' holds. It is used mainly by fumigation contractors whose staff are specially trained in safe procedures.

Routes of Absorption
This is by inhalation.

Pharmacology
The mode of action is not clearly defined but it is considered likely that methyl bromide binds to protein molecules, probably through the sulphydryl group, thus affecting intracellular metabolism. An alternative possibility is that an unknown metabolite is the toxin.

Toxic Effects
Methyl bromide is very toxic and causes (i) burns to the skin from contact with the liquid form, (ii) pulmonary oedema from inhalation of high concentrations of vapour and (iii) disorders of the central nervous system.

On the skin, splashes of methyl bromide in liquid form cause blisters — usually after a delay of several hours. They tend to be large, from the coalescence of numerous small vesicles, and surrounded by an area of redness and oedema. Itching is a constant symptom.

Methyl bromide in concentrations above 1 per cent by volume can be detected by smell and by the irritant effect of the mucous membranes of the eyes and the respiratory tract, thus giving warning of danger. Headache, soreness of the eyes, loss of appetite and abdominal discomfort lasting for a few days are the principal symptoms. There may also be peripheral paraesthesia affecting particularly the lower limbs and persisting sometimes for several months. Anuria may arise from renal tubular damage.

If a fumigant operator loses consciousness or is prevented from escaping from the fumes for some other reason, pulmonary oedema is likely to develop and may prove fatal. The onset of this complication may be delayed.

Disturbances of the central nervous system may follow exposure to low concentrations. Early symptoms, which are often ignored, are malaise, headache, smarting of the eyes and nausea. After a latent interval of some hours, more serious effects occur including difficulty in visual focussing, ataxia and incoherence, apathy, drowsiness, weakness (especially of the lower limbs) and convulsions.

Treatment
When skin contact has occurred the liquid should be washed off promptly and, as methyl bromide penetrates readily through any type of material, contaminated clothing, including boots, must be removed immediately. (Rubber absorbs and retains methyl bromide and should not be used for gloves or other items of personal protective equipment). With symptomatic treatment healing proceeds normally with little scarring. Dermatitis, characterised by a fine papular rash and a dry, cracked skin may result from repeated exposure to small amounts.

If inhalation has occurred the patient must be kept at rest and under observation, preferably in hospital, for at least forty-eight hours. The onset of pulmonary oedema is sudden and demands urgent treatment. Corticosteroids may be helpful.

Anuria calls for conventional support measures including haemodialysis.

Treatment of disturbances of the central nervous system is symptomatic. Depression, irritability, insomnia, visual disturbances and impairment of concentration may persist for months or even years and convalescence may be prolonged. It is unusual to find any objective evidence of central nervous system damage once the acute symptoms have subsided.

Laboratory Diagnosis

The measurement of blood bromide can be used to check and confirm exposure.

19(b). Carbon Tetrachloride

Uses
Carbon tetrachloride is seldom used alone as a fumigant but its penetrating powers are of value in the treatment of grain in deep-silo bins. High concentrations and long exposure are needed because the substance is not particularly toxic to insects. It is used more commonly in mixtures containing ethylene dichloride, ethylene dibromide or both, as a fire inhibiting agent and to increase penetration of the fumigants.

Route of Absorption
This is mainly by inhalation.

Pharmacology
Marked hepatoxic effects are induced whilst other tissues damaged include bone-marrow, brain, kidney and pancreas. Concentrations of vapour which cannot be readily detected may cause serious tissue damage.

Toxic Effects
In high doses the effect is narcotic causing headaches, dizziness, mental confusion, nausea and vomiting. Persons affected by the vapour have described the effects as similar to alcohol intoxication. Lassitude and anorexia may persist for several days.

After a latent period of 1-12 weeks these symptoms may be followed by renal failure and hepato-cellular jaundice. Effects may be more severe in persons who have been drinking alcohol in the immediate pre-exposure period and in habitual drinkers. There may be blurring of vision preceded by disturbance of colour vision.

Absorption through the skin also occurs and may cause similar systemic effects as well as a severe dermatitis, characterised by dry, fissured skin, due to the degreasing effect.

Treatment
Treatment is symptomatic. In acute poisoning the patient may be unconscious and in respiratory failure, and the usual supportive measures are then required. The patient must be kept under observation in hospital until it is certain that the kidneys and liver have not been affected. Renal failure may necessitate dialysis. For hepatic damage the patient should be referred, wherever possible, to a specialist gastro-enterologist.

Renal and hepatic function should be monitored in all cases where acute carbon tetrachloride poisoning is suspected and in those exposed repeatedly to concentrations causing less obvious symptoms such as persistent nausea, headache, lassitude and anorexia.

Laboratory Diagnosis
No specific test of carbon tetrachloride absorption is known.

19(c). Ethylene Dichloride
(1, 2-dichloroethane)

Uses
Ethylene dichloride is commonly used in a 3:1 or 1:1 mixture with carbon tetrachloride, the former for fumigating bagged products or grain in bulk storage less than 6 feet deep and the latter for grain deeper than this.

The presence of carbon tetrachloride reduces the risk of fire and increases the penetration of the fumigant

Route of Absorption
This is by inhalation.

Toxic Effects
Ethylene dichloride is a powerful narcotic and may cause renal and hepatic damage. In practice, however, effects on the kidney and liver have not been observed. Symptoms may occur as a result of its narcotic action and its irritant effect on the gastric mucosa. Loss of consciousness is rare but dizziness followed by frequent and persistent vomiting "similar to sea-sickness" is common. These effects usually last for a few hours only but may continue for several days.

Dermatitis can occur due to the degreasing effect on the skin.

Treatment
Treatment is symptomatic. It is important to enquire whether carbon tetrachloride was also used and, if so, to be on the alert for the symptoms and signs of poisoning with that substance.

Laboratory Diagnosis
No specific test is known.

19(d). Ethylene Dibromide
(1, 2-dibromoethane)

Uses
Ethylene dibromide is less volatile than carbon tetrachloride or ethylene dichloride. It is used, mixed with other substances, as a "spot" fumigant for treating machines and has the advantage that the degree of sealing required need not be so secure as for more volatile compounds. It is also used in bulk grain stores where, again, the low volatility increases effectiveness of treatment at the surface.

Route of Absorption
This is by inhalation.

Toxic Effects
Ethylene dibromide is irritating to the mucous membranes of the eyes and respiratory tract. The main effect observed in man is blistering following contact of the liquid with the skin. Extensive liver necrosis was found at necropsy in a woman, a known alcoholic, who had swallowed capsules containing ethylene dibromide. It was estimated that she had ingested 4.5 ml.

Treatment
Treatment is symptomatic. Splashes should be washed from the skin immediately and contaminated clothing removed. A check should be made on renal and hepatic function and, if indicated, appropriate treatment measures should be instituted accordingly.

Laboratory Diagnosis
No specific test is known.

19(e) Chloropicrin
(Trichloronitromethane)

Uses
Chloropicrin is used as a soil fumigant and disinfectant.

Route of Absorption
This is by inhalation.

Pharmacology
Chloropicrin is a powerful irritant of all body surfaces with which it comes into contact. In the presence of water and soil it breaks down to form hydrochloric acid, nitric acid and carbon dioxide. Phosgene may be formed in the presence of strong light.

It was used as a war gas in the 1914-1918 war and was known as "vomiting gas".

Toxic Effects
Its toxic effects are due to its irritant action. Marked irritation of the eyes occurs at a concentration of 1 ppm which acts as a warning of exposure. It is irritating to the eyes, skin and mucous membranes causing smarting of the eyes with lachrymation and blepharospasm; if inhaled, it causes bronchospasm, pulmonary oedema and vomiting.

Treatment
Treatment is symptomatic. The skin must be washed thoroughly after contaminated clothing has been removed. The effects on the respiratory system should be treated in the same way as for methyl bromide.

Laboratory Diagnosis
No specific test is known.

19(f). Phosphine
(From aluminium and magnesium phosphide preparations)

Uses
Aluminium or magnesium phosphide preparations are marketed in the form of tablets, pellets or as a powder in a paper sachet, with certain other ingredients intended to reduce the flammability of the phosphine gas which is produced by the action of moisture on the phosphide. These preparations are used principally for the fumigation of cereals and other raw foodstuffs but can be used for packaged foods and most materials infested with insect and mite pests if the residues of the phosphide preparations are removed and the treated materials are ventilated properly. Some products are used outdoors for the control of rats. The production of gas occurs over a period of several days and this period is extended where the temperature is below 10° C or if the relative humidity is low. Care must be taken over the disposal of the spent residues of all products.

Route of Absorption
Although the tablets, pellets or powder could be ingested, the principal hazard is by inhalation of the phosphine generated.

Pharmacology and Toxic Effects
Phosphine is a highly toxic gas which affects the gastro-intestinal and central nervous system. It has an odour similar to bad fish and this gives warning of the danger. Nausea, abdominal pain, vomiting and diarrhoea may be followed by ataxia, convulsions, coma and death within 24 hours. Other symptoms which have been described are vertigo, hyperacusis and burning substernal pain.

Treatment
There is no specific antidote and treatment is therefore symptomatic. If ingested, vomiting should be induced followed by gastric lavage.

Laboratory Diagnosis
No specific test is known.

19(g). Cyanides

Uses
Hydrogen cyanide is still used as a fumigant for some purposes. Cyanide gassing powders which liberate hydrogen cyanide in the presence of moisture are used for the control of rabbits and brown rats in agriculture and similar situations.

Routes of Absorption
Cyanide powders may be inadvertently or deliberately swallowed but the main risk is by inhalation of the hydrogen cyanide liberated.

Pharmacology
Cyanides conjugate with the enzyme ferricytochrome oxidase and thus prevent the transfer of oxygen from haemoglobin to tissue cells. Because the red cells remain oxygenated the blood, including venous blood, remains bright red until circulatory failure occurs.

Toxic Effects
The toxic effects are solely due to cellular hypoxia. Cyanides act rapidly and symptoms appear within a few seconds or minutes of inhaling the vapour or ingesting a cyanide compound. Death usually occurs rapidly unless immediate treatment is available. Occasionally recovery has occurred even when vital signs have been suppressed for some time.

Slight poisoning is characterised by a metallic taste, irritation of the nose and throat, dizziness, nausea, throbbing frontal headache, constriction of the chest, weakness of the limbs and a sensation of lack of air. Experienced operators recognise these symptoms and recover quickly on escaping to fresh air.

In more serious poisoning the patient rapidly becomes unconscious, develops Cheyne-Stokes breathing and may have convulsions. The pulse is thready and breathing becomes rapid and feeble before failing completely. Immediate treatment is essential to save life.

Treatment
If the patient is conscious, remove from the contaminated area, dispose of contaminated clothing and give symptomatic treatment. If cyanide has been swallowed induce vomiting, keep at rest, and observe for any signs indicative of a worsening of the patient's condition.

If the patient is unconcious, remove from the contaminated area and dispose of contaminated clothing. If breathing has stopped give artificial respiration, but avoid the "mouth-to-mouth" method.

Administer amyl nitrite capsules by inhalation one every 3 minutes until 6 have been given. Give oxygen when available.

For specific therapy two antidotes are available. These should be employed only when the signs of cyanide poisoning are observed and the diagnosis is not in doubt. In order of choice they are:

1. Cobalt EDTA (Kelocyanor)

    Inject intravenously 20 ml (1 ampoule) in two divided doses of 10 ml with an interval of 10 minutes between each dose. A second ampoule may be given if recovery is not complete.

2. Sodium nitrite/sodium thiosulphate

    Inject intravenously 0.3 g sodium nitrite dissolved in 10-15 ml sterile water at 2.5-5 ml per minute followed immediately by 25 g sodium thiosulphate in 50 ml sterile water injected slowly through the same needle. Both sodium nitrite and sodium thiosulphate are available as ready made injection solutions.

Appendix I

The Health and Safety (Agriculture) (Poisonous Substances) Regulations, 1975

These regulations place obligations on all users whether employed or self-employed of the 60 or so more toxic chemicals specified therein. Employers must provide prescribed protective clothing for their employees and ensure that it is worn for certain operations scheduled in the Regulations. Employees are required to wear the prescribed protective clothing. Self-employed persons must provide their own protective clothing and must wear it, in exactly the same circumstances as prescribed for employees.

Other requirements covered in the Regulations relate to:

a. the maximum number of hours operators may carry out scheduled operations;

b. the minimum age of operators working on operations covered by the Regulations;

c. extra precautions when working in greenhouses and livestock houses;

d. maintenance of protective clothing;

e. provision of washing facilities;

f. training and supervision of operators carrying out scheduled operations;

g. provision of drinking water vessels;

h. keeping of a register containing details of all scheduled operations carried out;

i. repairing of apparatus;

j. notification of sickness; the regulations require an employer to notify a Safety Inspector if he suspects that an employee may be suffering from poisoning by a specified substance; or if an employee is absent from work for more than three days and the employee worked for more than 60 hours in the preceding 14 days with dinoseb, dinoterb,

DNOC or medinoterb or their salts; or for more than 60 hours in the preceding 28 days with any other specified substance, unless the employer knows that the absence is not due to such poisoning. A self-employed person must notify an Inspector as soon as is reasonably practicable if he suspects that he may himself be suffering from poisoning by a specified substance.

The following chemicals are specified in the Health and Safety (Agriculture) (Poisonous Substances) Regulations 1975:—

1. **Dinitro Compounds**
    * dinoseb (DNBP) and its salts
    dinoterb and its salts
    * DNOC (DNC) and its salts
    medinoterb and its salts

2. **Organochlorine Compounds**
    endosulfan
    endrin

3. **Organophosphorus Compounds**
    amiton and its salts
    azinphos — ethyl
    azinphos — methyl
    chlorfenvinphos
    demephion
    demeton
    demeton — methyl
    demeton-S-methyl
    demeton-S-methyl sulphone
    dialifos
    * dichlorvos
    dimefox
    dioxathion
    disulfoton
    ethion
    fonofos
    mazidox
    mecarbam
    mephosfolan
    methidathion
    mevinphos
    mipafox
    omethoate
    oxydemeton-methyl
    parathion
    phenkapton

    phorate
    phosphamidon
    pirimiphos-ethyl
    schradan
    sulfotep
    TEPP
    thiometon
    thionazin
    triazophos
    vamidothion

4. **Fluoracetic Acid Derivatives**
   fluoracetamide

5. **Organomercury Compounds**
   Any used in aerosol form

6. **Arsenic Compounds**
   sodium arsenite
   potassium arsenite

7. **Organotin Compounds**
   fentin acetate
   fentin hydroxide

8. **Carbamates**
   aldicarb
   carbofuran
   methomyl
   oxamyl

9. **Soil Fumigants**
   *chloropicrin

10. **Miscellaneous Organic Compounds**
    cycloheximide
    drazoxolon
    endothal and its salts
    fenaminosulf
    fenazaflor
    formetanate
    *nicotine and its salts

*The Regulations do not apply to:

a. preparations used exclusively as insecticides which contain no more than 5 per cent by weight of dinoseb or DNOC or their respective salts;

b. preparations which contain no more than 5 per cent by weight of chloropicrin and no other specified substances;

c. preparations which contain no more than 7.5 per cent by weight of nicotine or its salts and no other specified substance;

d. aerosols containing not more than 1 per cent by weight of dichlorvos and no other specified substance;

e. materials impregnated with dichlorvos for slow release either into the air or into the digestive system of an animal.

Appendix II

Addresses and telephone numbers of Senior Employment Medical Advisers

Government Buildings
Kenton Bar
NEWCASTLE UPON TYNE
NE1 2YN
Tel: 0632 863411

8 St Pauls Street
LEEDS LS1 2LE
Tel: 0532 446191

14 Cardiff Road
LUTON
Beds LU1 1BB
Tel: 0582 34121

1 Long Lane
LONDON SE1 4PG
Tel: 01-407 8911

Intercity House (2nd Floor)
Mitchell Lane
Victoria Street
BRISTOL BS1 6AN
Tel: 0272 290681

McLaren Building
2 Masshouse Circus
Queensway
BIRMINGHAM B4 7NP
Tel: 021-236 5080

Quay House
Quay Street
MANCHESTER M3 3JE
Tel: 061-831 7111

Maritime House
1 Linton Road
BARKING
Essex IG11 8HF
Tel: 01-594 5522

Health & Safety Executive
Belford House
59 Belford Road
EDINBURGH EH4 3UE
Tel: 031-225 1313

Brunel House (13th Floor)
2 Fitzalan Road
CARDIFF CF2 1SH
Tel: 0222 497777

Department of Manpower Services
Netherleigh
Massey Avenue
BELFAST BT4 2JP
Tel: 0232 63244 — Ext 227

Appendix III
Cholinesterase Estimations

The following laboratories are able to carry out estimations relevant to pesticide poisoning of cholinesterase activity in heparinised whole blood. Red cell acetyl-cholinesterase activity can be measured as well as plasma cholinesterase activity.

Despatch Instructions
To comply with the Inland Postal regulations pathological specimens (blood, gastric contents, excreta, urine, etc) must be sent by letter post — **not** parcel post or sample post — packed in the manner described below, and conspicuously marked FRAGILE WITH CARE and bearing the words PATHOLOGICAL SPECIMEN (AGRICULTURAL POISON). A note should accompany each specimen giving (a) the name and age of the patient; (b) an indication of the degree of exposure to the poison, naming it if possible; and (c) details of any symptoms which may be referable to such exposure.

Specimens must be enclosed in a receptacle, hermetically sealed or otherwise securely closed, and this receptacle must itself be placed in a strong wooden or metal case, or an alternative container approved by the Post Office in such a way that it cannot shift about, and with a sufficient quantity of some absorbent material (such as sawdust or cotton wool) packed about the receptacle to prevent absolutely any possible leakage from the package in the event of damage to the receptacle. Such specimens — which are otherwise prohibited for transmission by post — may be sent for medical examination or analysis only to a recognised medical laboratory or institute (whether or not belonging to a public health authority) or to a qualified medical practitioner. Any packet containing specimens, found in the parcel post or sample post, or found in the letter post not packed and marked as directed, will be at once stopped and destroyed with all the wrappings and enclosures. Anyone sending by post such a specimen (described in the regulations as "deleterious liquid or substance") other than as provided for by the regulations is liable to prosecution.

Receptacles used by a laboratory or institute which are not cleared for transmission by post must be submitted to Postal Headquarters (PMk 1) St Martin's-le-Grand, London EC1A 1HQ to ensure that they comply with the regulations.

Regional Health Authority Laboratories

England

Northern Region
Department of Pathology,
Newcastle General Hospital,
Westgate Road,
Newcastle upon Tyne, NE4 6BE
Tel: 0632 738811
(during normal working hours)

Department of Pathology,
Middlesbrough General Hospital,
Ayresome Green,
Middlesbrough,
Cleveland TS5 5AZ
Tel: 0642 81333
(during normal working hours)

Yorkshire Region
Department of Pathology,
Hull Royal Infirmary,
Anlaby Road,
Hull HU3 2JZ
Tel: 0482 28541

Trent Region
Department of Chemical Pathology,
University Hospital,
Queen's Medical Centre,
Nottingham NG7 2UH.
Tel: 0602 700111

East Anglian Region
Department of Clinical Chemistry,
Peterborough District Hospital,
Thorpe Road,
Peterborough PE3 6DA.
Tel: 0733 67451

North East Thames Region
Department of Pathology,
Essex County Hospital,
Lexden Road,
Colchester,
Essex CO3 3NB.
Tel: 0206 69244

Department of Pathology,
Chase Farm Hospital,
The Ridgeway,
Enfield,
Middlesex EN2 8JL.
Tel: 366 6600

North West Thames Region
Department of Clinical Chemistry,
Watford General Hospital,
Peace Memorial Wing,
Rickmansworth Road,
Watford,
Herts. WD1 7HH.
Tel: 0923 25611

Department of Clinical Chemistry,
Barnet General Hospital,
Wellhouse Lane,
Barnet,
Herts. EN5 3DJ.
Tel: 01 440 5111

Biochemistry Department,
Edgware General Hospital,
Edgware,
Middx. HA8 0AD.
Tel: 01 952 2381

Chemical Pathology Department,
Central Middlesex Hospital,
Acton Lane,
NW10 7NS.
Tel: 01 965 5733

Chemical Pathology Department,
St Albans City Hospital,
Normandy Road,
St Albans,
Herts. AL3 5PN.
Tel: 56 66122

Department of Clinical Enzymology,
Hammersmith Hospital,
Ducane Road,
W12 0HS.
Tel: 01 743 2030

93

Department of Biochemistry,
Hillingdon Hospital,
Uxbridge,
Middx. UB8 3NN.
Tel: 0895 38282

Department of Biochemistry,
Lister Hospital,
Coreys Mill Lane,
Stevenage,
Herts. SG1 4AB.
Tel: 0438 4333

Chemical Pathology Department,
Bedford General Hospital,
Kimbolton Road,
Bedford, MK40 2NU.
Tel: 0234 55122

Department of Biochemistry,
Luton and Dunstable Hospital,
Lewsey Road,
Luton, LU4 0DT.
Tel: 0582 53211

South East Thames Region

Group Laboratory,
Lewisham Hospital,
High Street,
Lewisham,
London SE13 6LH.
Tel: 01 690 4311

South West Thames Region

Group Laboratory,
Mayday Hospital,
Mayday Road,
Thornton Heath,
Surrey, CR4 7YE.
Tel: 01 684 699

Group Laboratory,
St Luke's Hospital,
Warren Road,
Guildford,
Surrey, GU1 3NT.
Tel: 0483 71122

Area Laboratory,
West Park Hospital,
Epsom,
Surrey.
Tel: 78 27811

Department of Pathology,
Ashford Hospital,
London Road,
Ashford,
Middx. TW15 3AA.
Tel: 69 51188

St Helier Hospital,
Wrythe Lane,
Carshalton,
Surrey, SM5 1AA.
Tel: 01 641 4011

Worthing Hospital,
Lynhurst Road,
Worthing,
Sussex.
Tel: 0903 205111

Oxford Region

Nuffield Department of Clinical
  Biochemistry,
Radcliffe Infirmary,
Woodstock Road,
Oxford, OX2 6HE.
Tel: 0865 49891

Kettering General Hospital,
Rothwell Road,
Kettering,
Northants. NN16 8UZ.
Tel: 0536 81141

Horton General Hospital,
Oxford Road,
Banbury,
Oxon, OX16 9AL.
Tel: 0295 4521

Northampton General Hospital,
Billing Road,
Northampton, NN1 5BD.
Tel: 0604 34700
(during normal working hours)

Royal Berkshire Hospital,
London Road,
Reading, RG1 5AN.
Tel: 0734 85111

South Western Region
Area Department of Pathology,
Church Lane,
Heavitree,
Exeter,
Devon.
Tel: 0392 77833

West Midlands Region
Department of Pathology,
Warwick General Hospital,
Lakin Road,
Warwick,
Warwickshire.
Tel: 0926 45321

Department of Pathology,
Worcester Royal Infirmary,
Ronkswood Branch,
Newton Road,
Worcester, WR5 1HN.
Tel: 0905 356123

Department of Pathology,
Dudley Road Hospital,
Dudley Road,
Birmingham, B18 7QH.
Tel: 021 554 3801

Department of Clinical Chemistry,
Burton-on-Trent General Hospital,
New Street,
Burton-on-Trent,
Staffs. DE14 3QH.
Tel: 0283 6334

Department of Biochemistry,
Coventry and Warwickshire Hospital,
Stoney Stanton Road,
Coventry, CV1 4FH.
Tel: 0203 24055
(during normal working hours)

Department of Clinical Chemistry,
New Cross Hospital,
Wolverhampton, WV10 0QP.
Tel: 0902 73255
(during normal working hours)

Department of Pathology,
County Hospital,
Hereford, HR1 2ER.
Tel: 0432 68161

Department of Pathology,
East Birmingham Hospital,
Bordesley,
Green East,
Birmingham, B9 5ST.
Tel: 021 772 4311

Department of Pathology,
Good Hope General Hospital,
Rectory Road,
Sutton Coldfield,
West Midlands, B75 7RR.
Tel: 021 378 2211

North Western Region
Department of Clinical Pathology,
Manchester Royal Infirmary,
Oxford Road,
Manchester, M13 9WL.
Tel: 061 273 3300
(during normal working hours)

Department of Pathology,
Burnley General Hospital,
Casterton Avenue,
Burnley,
Lancs. BB10 2PQ.
Tel: 0282 25071
(during normal working hours)

Department of Pathology,
Bury General Hospital,
Walmersley Road,
Bury, BL9 6PG.
Tel: 061 764 0511
(during normal working hours)

Department of Pathology,
Stepping Hill Hospital,
Poplar Grove,
Stockport, SK2 7JE.
Tel: 061 483 1010
(during normal working hours)

Mersey Region
Department of Pathology,
Macclesfield Hospital
(West Park Branch),
Prestbury Road,
Macclesfield,
Cheshire, SK10 3BL.
Tel: 0625 21000

Wessex Region

Department of Pathology,
Royal Hampshire County Hospital,
Romsey Road,
Winchester,
Hants. SO22 5DG.
Tel: 0962 63535

Department of Pathology,
Salisbury General Hospital,
General Infirmary Branch,
Fisherton Street,
Salisbury,
Wilts. SP2 7SX.
Tel: 0772 6212

Department of Pathology,
Royal Victoria Hospital,
Shelley Road,
Boscombe,
Bournemouth, BH1 4JG.
Tel: 0202 35201

County Laboratory,
Glyde Path Road,
Dorchester,
Dorset, DT1 1XD.
Tel: 0305 67341

Department of Chemical Pathology,
Southampton General Hospital,
Tremona Road,
Shirley,
Southampton,
Hants. SO9 4XY.
Tel: 0703 777222

Wales

Department of Pathology,
Caernarvon and Anglesey General
 Hospital,
Bangor Gwynedd, LL57 2HW.
Tel: 0248 53321
*(usually during normal working
hours, but 24 hour service available
if deemed necessary after
consultation.)*

Biochemistry Department,
Llandough Hospital,
Penarth,
South Glamorgan, CF6 1XX.
Tel: 0222 708601
*(usually during normal working
hours, but 24 hour service available
if necessary.)*

Department of Pathology,
Royal Gwent Hospital,
Cardiff Road,
Newport,
Gwent, NPT 2UB.
Tel: 0633 52244
(during normal working hours)

Biochemistry Department,
Nevill Hall Hospital,
Abergavenny,
Gwent, NP7 7EG.
Tel: 0873 2091
(during normal working hours)

Biochemistry Department,
Neath General Hospital,
Neath,
West Glamorgan, SA11 2LQ.
Tel: 0639 4161
(during normal working hours)

Department of Pathology,
Withybush Hospital,
Haverfordwest,
Dyfed, SA1 1PG.
Tel: 0437 4545
*(during normal working hours
but 24 hour service available if
necessary)*

Biochemistry Department,
Bronglais General Hospital,
Aberystwyth,
Dyfed, SY23 2EF.
Tel: 0970 3131
(during normal working hours)

Biochemistry Department,
Ysbyty Glan Clwyd,
Bodelwyddan Nr. Rhyl,
Clwyd, LL18 5UJ.
Tel: 0745 583910
(during normal working hours but 24 hour service available in exceptional circumstances; eg known exposure to spray).

Department of Pathology,
Llanelli General Hospital,
Marble Hall Road,
Llanelli, SA15 1NL.
Tel: 05542 4961
(during normal working hours)

Biochemistry Department,
West Wales General Hospital,
Glangwilli,
Carmarthen,
Dyfed.
Tel: 0267 5151

Department of Pathology,
Bridgend General Hospital,
Quarella Road,
Bridgend,
Mid Glamorgan, CF31 1JS.
Tel: 0656 62166
(during normal working hours)

Biochemistry Department,
Maelor General Hospital,
Croesnewydd,
Wrexham,
Clwyd, LL13 7TD.
Tel: 0978 53153
(during normal working hours)

Scotland

Chemical Pathology Department,
Aberdeen Royal Infirmary,
Foresterhill,
Aberdeen, AB9 2ZB.
Tel: 0224 681818

Department of Biochemical Medicine,
Ninewells Hospital,
Dundee, DD2 1UB.
Tel: 0382 60111

Biochemistry Department,
Regional Laboratory,
Raigmore Hospital,
Inverness, IV2 3UJ.
Tel: 0463 34151

Fife District Laboratory,
Victoria Hospital,
Hayfield Road,
Kirkcaldy,
Fife, KY2 5AH.
Tel: 0592 61155

Department of Clinical Chemistry,
Bangour General Hospital,
Broxburn,
West Lothian, EH52 6LR.
Tel: 050 681 334

Department of Clinical Chemistry,
Western General Hospital,
Crewe Road,
Edinburgh, EH4 3XU.
Tel: 031 332 2525

Department of Clinical Chemistry,
Royal Infirmary of Edinburgh,
Lauriston Place,
Edinburgh, EH3 9YW.
Tel: 031 229 2477

Biochemistry Department,
Dumfries and Galloway Royal Infirmary,
Nithbank,
Dumfries, DG1 2SA.
Tel: 0387 3151

Biochemistry Department,
Ballochmyle Hospital,
Mauchline,
Ayrshire, KA5 6LQ.
Tel: 0290 51281/51581

Biochemistry Department,
Glasgow Royal Infirmary,
84 Castle Street,
Glasgow, G4 0SF.
Tel: 041 552 3535

Biochemistry Department,
Gartnavel General Hospital,
1053 Great Western Road,
Glasgow, G12 0XH.
Tel: 041 334 6241

Biochemistry Department,
Hawkhead Hospital,
Hawkhead Road,
Paisley, PA2 7BZ.
Tel: 041 889 8151

Northern Ireland

Royal Victoria Hospital Laboratory,
Institute of Pathology,
Grosvenor Road,
Belfast, BT12 6BA.
Tel: 0232 40503

The Laboratories,
Belfast City Hospital,
Lisburn Road,
Belfast, BT9 7AD.
Tel: 0232 29241

Appendix IV

Centres holding supplies of Pralidoxime — P2S

(A 24 hour service is maintained. When contacting a listed hospital at night ask for the Nursing Superintendent or Medical Officer in Charge unless otherwise stated here).

England

Northern Region

1. The Pharmacy Department
   Cumberland Infirmary
   CARLISLE CA2 7HY
   Tel. 0228 23444

2. The Principal Pharmacist
   Newcastle General Hospital
   Westgate Road
   NEWCASTLE-UPON-TYNE NE4 6BE
   Tel. 0632 738811

3. The District Pharmaceutical Officer
   Darlington Memorial Hospital
   Hollyhurst Road
   DARLINGTON
   Co Durham DL3 6HS
   Tel. 0325 60100

Yorkshire Region

4. The District Pharmaceutical Officer
   Castle Hill Hospital
   Castle Road
   COTTINGHAM
   N Humberside HU16 5JQ
   Tel. 0482 659331

5. The Principal Pharmacist
   Leeds General Infirmary
   St George Street
   LEEDS LS1 3EX
   Tel. 0532 32799

6. The Pharmaceutical Officer
   Hull Royal Infirmary
   Anlaby Road
   HULL HU3 2JZ
   Tel. 0482 28541

Trent Region

7. The Principal Pharmacist
   Nottingham City Hospital
   Hucknall Road
   Nottingham NG5 1PB
   Tel. 0602 608111

8. The Senior Casualty Officer
   The Casualty Department
   County Hospital
   Sewell Road
   Lincoln LN2 5Q7
   Tel. 0522 29921 Ext. 222

9. The Principal Pharmacist
   Pharmacy Department
   Royal Hallamshire Hospital
   Glossop Road
   Sheffield S10 2JF
   Tel. 0742 26484

10. The Pharmacy
    Pilgrim Hospital
    Sibsey Road
    Boston
    Lincolnshire PE21 9QT
    Tel. 0205 64801

11. The District Pharmaceutical Officer
    University Hospital
    Queen's Medical Centre
    Nottingham NG7 2UH
    Tel. 0602 70111

12. Grantham & Kesteven General Hospital
    Manthorpe Road
    Grantham
    Lincs.
    Tel. 0476 5232

13. Skegness & District Hospital
    Dorothy Avenue
    Skegness
    Lincs. PE25 2BS
    Tel. 0754 2401

14. Holbeach Hospital
    Boston Road
    Holbeach
    Lincs. PE12 8AQ
    Tel. 0406 22283

15. Johnson Hospital
    Priory Road
    Spalding
    Lincs. PE11 2XD
    Tel. 0775 2386/7

East Anglian Region

16. The Director
    Regional Transfusion and Immuno-Haematology Centre
    Long Road
    Cambridge CB2 2PT
    Tel. 0223 45921

17. The District Pharmaceutical Officer
    Norfolk and Norwich Hospital
    St Stephen's Road
    Norwich
    Norfolk NR1 3SR
    Tel. 0603 28377 Ext. 237

18. The Pharmacy
    Peterborough General Hospital
    Thorpe Road
    Peterborough PE3 6DA
    Tel. 0733 67451 Ext. 389

19. The Pharmacy
    Ipswich Hospital
    Anglesea Road Wing
    Anglesea Road
    Ipswich IP1 3PY
    Tel. 0473 212477 Ext. 263

20. The District Pharmaceutical Officer
    Queen Elizabeth Hospital
    Gayton Road
    Kings Lynn
    Norfolk PE30 4ET
    Tel. 0603 28377

North West Thames Region

21. The Chief Pharmacist
    Edgware General Hospital
    Edgware
    Middlesex HA8 0AD
    Tel. 01 952 2381

22. The Principal Pharmacist
    Bedford General Hospital
    (South Wing)
    Kempston Road
    Bedford MK42 9DJ
    Tel. 0234 55122

23. The Principal Pharmacist
    Luton and Dunstable Hospital
    Dunstable Road
    Luton
    Beds. LU4 0DZ
    Tel. 0582 53211
24. Pharmacy Department
    West Middlesex Hospital
    Twickenham Road
    Isleworth
    Middlesex TW7 6AF
    Tel. 01 560 2121

North East Thames Region

25. The Microbiologist
    North Middlesex Hospital
    Silver Street
    London N18 1QX
    Working Hours: 807 3071 Ext. 472
    Other Times: 807 3071 (contact Microbiologist on-call via Switchboard)
26. The Pathology Department
    Chelmsford and Essex Hospital
    London Road
    Chelmsford
    Essex CM2 0QH
    Working Hours: 0245 355139 or 355140
    Other Times: 0245 354467 (ask for duty MLSO)
27. The Principal Pharmacist
    Oldchurch Hospital
    Romford
    Essex RM7 0BE
    Working Hours: 70 46090 Ext. 3321
    Other Times: 70 46090 Ext. 3252 (Ward D2)

South East Thames Region

28. Principal Pharmacist
    Kent and Sussex Hospital
    Mount Ephraim
    Tunbridge Wells
    Kent TN4 8AT
    Tel. 0892 26111 Ext. 6
29. Principal Pharmacist
    Kent and Canterbury Hospital
    Ethelbert Road
    Canterbury
    Kent CT1 3NG
    Tel. 0227 66877

30. The Director
    The Poisons Unit
    New Cross Hospital
    Avonley Road
    London SE14 5ER
    Tel. 01 407 7600
31. The District Pharmaceutical Officer
    Accident Unit
    Royal Sussex County Hospital
    Eastern Road
    Brighton BN2 5BE
    Tel. 0273 606611

South West Thames Region

32. The Director
    South London Transfusion Centre
    75 Cranmer Terrace
    Tooting
    London SW17 0RB
    Tel. 01 672 8501/7
33. The District Pharmaceutical Officer
    Epsom District Hospital
    Dorking Road
    Epsom
    Surrey KT18 7EG
    Tel. 78 26100

Oxford Region

34. The District Pharmaceutical Officer
    Northampton General Hospital
    Billing Road
    Northampton NN1 5BD
    Tel. 0604 34700
35. The District Pharmaceutical Officer
    Royal Berkshire Hospital
    London Road
    Reading
    Berks. RG1 5AN
    Tel. 0734 875111
36. The Chief Pharmacist
    Wexham Park Hospital
    Wexham
    Slough
    Berks. SL2 4HL
    Tel. 0753 34567

South Western Region

37. The Officer in Charge
    Accident and Emergency Department
    Royal Devon and Exeter Hospital
    Barrack Road
    Exeter
    Devon EX2 5DW
    Tel. 0392 77833 Ext. 2207

38. The Officer in Charge
    Accident and Emergency Department
    Plymouth General Hospital (Freedom Fields)
    Plymouth
    Devon PLA 7JJ
    Tel. 0752 668080

39. Area Pharmaceutical Department (Out of hours — On-call pharmacist)
    Royal Cornwall Hospital
    Treliske Branch
    Truro
    Cornwall TR1 3LJ
    Tel. 0872 74242

40. The Nurse in Charge
    Accident Department
    Southmead General Hospital
    Westbury on Trym
    Bristol BS10 5NB
    Tel. 0272 505050 Ext. 303

41. The Pharmacy Department (Out of hours — On-call pharmacist)
    Taunton and Somerset Hospital (Musgrove Park Branch)
    Taunton
    Somerset TA1 5DA
    Tel. 0823 73444

West Midlands Region

42. The Principal Pharmacist
    Staffordshire General Infirmary
    Foregate Street
    Stafford ST16 2PA
    Tel. 0785 58251

43. The Principal Pharmacist
    Dudley Road Hospital
    Birmingham B18 7QH
    Tel. 021 554 3801

44. The Medical Officer on Duty
    Accident and Emergency Department
    General Hospital
    Nelson Street
    Hereford HR1 2PA
    Tel. 0432 2561

45. The Consultant Surgeon in Charge
    Accident and Emergency Department
    Worcester Royal Infirmary
    Castle Street Branch
    Castle Street
    Worcester WR1 3AS
    Tel. 0905 27122

46. The District Pharmaceutical Officer
    Worcester Royal Infirmary
    Ronkswood Branch
    Newton Road
    Worcester WR5 1HH
    Tel. 0905 356123

47. The District Pharmaceutical Officer
    Royal Shrewsbury Hospital
    Copthorne North
    Mytton Oak Road
    Shrewsbury
    Salop SY3 8XF
    Tel. 0743 52244

48. The Pharmacist in Charge
    North Staffordshire Royal Infirmary
    Princes Road
    Hartshill
    Stoke-on-Trent
    Staffs. ST4 7EN
    Tel. 0782 49144

49. The Principal Pharmacist
    Burton-on-Trent General Hospital
    New Street
    Burton-on-Trent
    Staffs. DE14 3QH
    Tel. 0283 63334

North Western Region

50. The Principal Pharmacist
    Manchester Royal Infirmary
    Oxford Road
    Manchester M13 9WL
    Tel. 061 273 3300

51. The Group Pharmacist
    Royal Preston Hospital
    PO Box 66
    Sharoe Green Lane
    Fulwood
    Preston PR2 4HT
    Tel. 0772 716565

Mersey Region

52. The Pharmacy Department
    Walton Hospital
    Rice Lane
    Liverpool L9 1AE
    Tel. 051 525 3611

53. The Pharmacy Department
    Warrington General Hospital
    Lovely Lane
    Warrington
    Cheshire WA5 1QG
    Tel. 0925 35911

54. The Pharmacy Department
    Chester Royal Infirmary
    St Martin's Way
    Chester CH1 2AZ
    Tel. 0244 315500

Wessex Region

55. The Staff Pharmacist
    Royal Portsmouth Hospital
    Commercial Road
    Portsmouth
    Hants. PO1 4BS
    Tel. 0705 22281

56. The Principal Pharmacist
    Southampton General Hospital
    Tremona Road
    Shirley
    Southampton
    Hants. SO9 4XY
    Tel. 0703 777222

57. The Pharmacy
    Queen Alexandra Hospital
    Cosham
    Portsmouth PO6 3LY
    Tel. 0705 379451 Ext. 2105

58. The District Pharmaceutical Officer
    Royal Victoria Hospital
    Shelley Road
    Boscombe
    Dorset BH1 4JG
    Tel. 0202 35201

59. The Principal Pharmacist
    Basingstoke District Hospital
    Aldermaston Road
    Basingstoke RG24 9NA
    Tel. 0256 3202

60. The Area Pharmaceutical Officer
    Princess Margaret Hospital
    Obus Road
    Swindon
    Wiltshire SN1 4JU
    Tel. 0793 36231 Ext. 387

Wales

61. The Principal Pharmacist
    Cardiff Royal Infirmary
    Newport Road
    Cardiff CF2 1SZ
    Tel. 0222 33101

62. The Principal Pharmacist
    Caernarvon and Anglesey General Hospital
    Bangor
    Gwynedd LL57 2HW
    Tel. 0248 53321

63. The Principal Pharmacist
    Maelor General Hospital
    Croesnewydd Road
    Wrexham
    Clwyd LL13 7TD
    Tel. 0978 53153

64. The Principal Pharmacist
    West Wales General Hospital
    Glangwili
    Dyfed SA31 2AF
    Tel. 0267 5151

65. The Principal Pharmacist
    Bronglais General Hospital
    Caradog Road
    Aberystwyth
    Dyfed SY23 1ER
    Tel. 0970 3131/7

66. The Principal Pharmacist
    Ysbyty Glan Clwyd
    Bodelwyddan
    Rhyl
    Clwyd
    Tel. 0745 583910

67. The Principal Pharmacist
    Royal Gwent Hospital
    Cardiff Road
    Newport
    Gwent NPT 2UB
    Tel. 0633 52244

68. The Principal Pharmacist
    Brecon War Memorial Hospital
    Cerrigcochion Road
    Brecon
    Powys LD3 7NS
    Tel. 0874 2443

Scotland

69. The District Pharmaceutical Officer
    Pharmacy Department
    Law Hospital
    Carluke
    Lanarkshire ML8 5ER
    Tel. 06983 71100

70. The District Pharmaceutical Officer
    Pharmacy Department
    Bridge of Earn Hospital
    Bridge of Earn
    Perthshire PH2 9AQ
    Tel. 0738 81 331/7

71. The Principal Pharmacist (Sterile Products)
    Pharmaceutical Department
    Royal Infirmary of Edinburgh
    Lauriston Place
    Edinburgh EH3 9YW
    Tel. 031 229 2477

72. The Chief Administrative Pharmaceutical Officer
    Pharmacy Department
    Dumfries and Galloway Royal Infirmary
    (New District General Hospital)
    Bankend Road
    Dumfries DG1 4AP
    Tel. 0387 3151

73. Senior Medical Laboratory Scientist
    Clinical Laboratory
    Caithness Central Hospital
    Wick
    Caithness KW1 5LA
    Tel. 0955 2261

74. The District Pharmaceutical Officer
    Department of Pharmacy
    Aberdeen Royal Infirmary
    Foresterhill
    Aberdeen AB9 2ZB
    Tel. 0224 23423

75. The Chief Administrative Pharmaceutical Officer
Pharmaceutical Department
Peel Hospital
Galashiels
Selkirkshire TD1 3LQ
Tel. 0896 2295

76. The District Pharmaceutical Officer
Pharmacy Department
Raigmore Hospital
Inverness IV2 3UJ
Tel. 0463 34151

77. Chief Administrative Medical Officer
Shetland Health Board
28 Burgh Road
Lerwick
Shetland ZE1 0QP
Tel. 0595 2945

78. The Staff Pharmacist
Pharmaceutical Department
Ninewells Hospital
Ninewells
Dundee DD2 1UB
Tel. 0382 60111

Northern Ireland

79. District Pharmaceutical Officer
Pharmaceutical Department
Altnagelvin Hospital
Londonderry BT47 1JB
Tel. 0504 45171

80. District Pharmaceutical Officer
Royal Victoria Hospital
Grosvenor Road
Belfast BT12 6BA
Tel. 0232 40503

81. Area Pharmaceutical Officer
Pharmaceutical Department
Craigavon Area Hospital
68 Lurgan Road
Portadown
Craigavon
Co Armagh BT63 5QQ
Tel. 0762 34444

82. Area Pharmaceutical Officer
Waveney Hospital
Ballymena
Co Antrim BT42 6HR
Tel. 0266 3377

Printed in the UK for HMSO
Dd 736666 C415 3/83